PRACTICAL
PATIENT LITERACY
THE MEDAGOGY MODEL

Melissa N. Stewart, DNP, RN, CPE
Faculty
School of Nursing
Our Lady of the Lake College
Baton Rouge, Louisiana

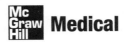 **Medical**

New York   Chicago   San Francisco   Lisbon   London   Madrid   Mexico City
Milan   New Delhi   San Juan   Seoul   Singapore   Sydney   Toronto

The McGraw·Hill Companies

Practical Patient Literacy: The Medagogy Model

Copyright © 2012 by Melissa N. Stewart. Published by The McGraw-Hill Companies, Inc. All rights reserved. Printed in the United States of America. Except as permitted under the United States Copyright Act of 1976, no part of this publication may be reproduced or distributed in any form or by any means, or stored in a data base or retrieval system, without the prior written permission of the publisher.

1 2 3 4 5 6 7 8 9 0   DOC/DOC   16 15 14 13 12

ISBN 978-0-07-176131-4
MHID 0-07-176131-4

This book was set in Plantin by Thomson Digital.
The editors were Joseph Morita, Robert Pancotti, and Catherine A. Johnson.
The production supervisor was Jeffrey Herzich.
Project management was provided by Mala Arora, Thomson Digital.
The cover designer was Joanne Lee.
RR Donnelley was printer and binder.

This book is printed on acid-free paper.

Library of Congress Cataloging-in-Publication Data
Stewart, Melissa N.
  Practical patient literacy : the medagogy model / Melissa N. Stewart.
    p. ; cm.
  Includes bibliographical references and index.
  ISBN-13: 978-0-07-176131-4 (pbk. : alk. paper)
  ISBN-10: 0-07-176131-4 (pbk. : alk. paper)
  I. Title.
  [DNLM: 1. Health Literacy—methods. 2. Patient Education as
Topic—methods. WA 590]
  610.73—dc23

                                                          2011035319

McGraw-Hill books are available at special quantity discounts to use as premiums and sales promotions, or for use in corporate training programs. To contact a representative, please e-mail us at bulksales@mcgraw-hill.com.

This book is dedicated to my family, Steve, Taylor, and Ashton Stewart: thank you for the wings. And to the memory of my precious parents, Svend and Phyllis Nielsen: thank you for the wind. May the information in this book bless and empower numerous lives.

Contents

Foreword

As a patient, am I learning what I need to know to make an informed decision on things that impact my health? The short answer is no, not adequately. As a father and husband, do I know what I need to know to keep my family well? I pitch in, but the truth is that my sweet wife takes the lion's share of responsibility here. As a healthcare administrator, do I think that standardizing the process and tools to better educate patients can positively impact our health? Definitely, I do. As a Six Sigma Black Belt, do I know how important it is to have a valid and reliable process in order to produce optimal results? I must admit that I do. So this begs the question—Can we design a more reliable patient education process that delivers better results? Unequivocally, I believe that we can vastly improve patient outcomes through standardizing the methodology used for patient education.

Melissa Stewart's pioneering framework around patient education offers structure to the patient education process, which has been grossly nonexistent in healthcare prior to her work. Her Medagogy Conceptual Framework breaks new ground by applying theories that are commonly practiced in traditional educational settings but are less customary in healthcare settings where patient information is perpetually dispersed. Dr. Stewart's work offers resolution in addressing the complex problem of health literacy through a strategy that is simple and effective. I believe that the future of healthcare revolves around our ability to empower patients to make good decisions, and Dr. Stewart's model allows for that to be done by all healthcare providers in a coordinated way that builds knowledge and leads to patient empowerment.

Melissa Stewart's work greatly contributed to the success of eQHealth Solutions' Care Transitions project, which is part of our contract as the Medicare Quality Improvement Organization for Louisiana. eQHealth engaged patients in knowledge-growth using Dr. Stewart's Medagogy Framework, yielding results that demonstrated a substantial decrease in 30-day hospital readmission rates. As a contractor for Medicare, we have access to nationally recognized experts to achieve success in improving Quality of Care, and Melissa Stewart's subject-matter expertise is ingrained throughout our Care Transitions work. We trained our staff of coaches, both clinical and non-clinical personnel, on the Medagogy Framework (inclusive of the PITS Model and the UPP Tool), and incorporated Stewart's framework throughout our patient coaching work.

This was not necessarily embraced or welcomed at first by our staff until they realized the power of the Medagogy process and the effect it has on patient knowledge-gain and ultimately on patients' health. Our staff then became energized around applying Stewart's framework in a systematic way to improve care, and they began to unlock the potential impact with each patient coached.

Those who know Melissa Stewart well can certainly attest to her unbridled passion for patient education, which is quite evident in her work. She is an outstanding college educator with a mission to educate her students in a comprehensive way by challenging them to master the concepts as well as the application. This book is a good representation of Dr. Stewart's passion, knowledge, and teaching style.

Dr. Stewart's work provides hope for successful health gains, health maintenance, and health prevention through shared knowledge in the patient–provider relationship while re-humanizing the care process so that each unique patient's personal health goals are addressed. As a patient, father, and healthcare administrator dedicated to improving quality, I believe that her work will greatly contribute to improving our effectiveness as healthcare providers and empowering patients to make intentional decisions that will collectively improve our health.

Scott M. Flowers, MHA, MBA, CPHQ
Lean Six Sigma Black Belt
Executive Director
Louisiana QIO
Vice President of Professional Services
Thibodaux Regional Medical Center

Preface

> *"It was the best of times, it was the worst of times, it was the age of wisdom, it was the age of foolishness, it was the epoch of belief, it was the epoch of incredulity, it was the season of Light, it was the season of Darkness, it was the spring of hope, it was the winter of despair, we had everything before us, we had nothing before us..."*

> *Charles Dickens*
> *A Tale of Two Cities*

Medagogy

The Medagogy conceptual framework has been a work of the heart, a decade in the making. Before health literacy was a common term, as a healthcare provider my curiosity had already started questioning why patients were constantly returning to access points of care as if they were in a frequent-flyer rewards program.

The revolving door associated with recidivism continued as I pursued higher educational opportunities. In my graduate studies, I was exposed to learning and teaching theory that piqued my interest in patient teaching and the learning process. In my master's degree studies, the PITS model served as the focus of my thesis. Simplicity of the model, coupled with the practicality of its use, stimulated appeals from colleagues for continued development and work in health literacy and patient education.

Care Transitions Success

Though new to many, the Medagogy model is not new to healthcare. The Medagogy model played an integral role in the success of the nationally recognized Centers for Medicaid and Medicare Systems' (CMS) Care Transitions pilot. From coach to physician, all healthcare providers in the award-winning pilot were trained in the Medagogy model. The ease of application and implementation within a practice setting made Medagogy the perfect fit for Care Transitions. Since the success of the pilot, the Medagogy model has been cited as the process that every healthcare provider should know and be held to for patient education.

This book is written for healthcare providers and is designed to walk the reader through empirically proven theoretical educational, psychological, and behavioral theories and neurocognitive science of learning, which serve as the foundational support for the Medagogy structure. As the reader progresses through the book, fundamental parts of the Medagogy model will be introduced individually. The culmination of this journey is met when all of the parts are presented together in a global overview of the Medagogy model followed by the Understanding Personal Perspective (UPP) tool.

The Center of It All: The Patient

The Medagogy model serves to bridge the information gap between patients and healthcare providers. Integral parts of the Medagogy model, the health informational seasons, the patient education hierarchy, the PITS model, and the UPP tool serve to aid healthcare providers, individually and jointly, in their patient educational efforts.

Medagogy is built on empirically proven, age-old teaching, learning, psychological, and behavioral principles and theories. Replication of academic tools such as teaching plans, homework, and a report card system offer socially acceptable and familiar instruments known to aid in knowledge progression. The interdisciplinary synergism of information disbursement to patients as they progress through the healthcare continuum presents the opportunity for shared knowledge to occur in the patient–provider relationship.

Technology and advancements in genetics have offered healthcare a glimpse into what could be the best of times in our industry. Every day, people's lives are being saved through the miracle of modern medicine. Unfortunately, a closer look reveals that healthcare also is facing the worst of times. Life is expensive and healthy living is even more costly. The lives being saved and the knowledge being used to save them are leaving a strong fiscal imprint on our economy that reaches into each and every household.

Preventable errors and fragmented care are challenging our healthcare delivery system into a new era, where quality and outcomes determine provider reimbursement. This new day in healthcare offers the promise of change. Alterations will occur in the dynamics among all players involved from provider to patient.

Strengthening the Patient–Provider Bond

Providers will need to seek out strong relationships with the consumers of their services—both patients and other healthcare professionals. Nonchalant, passive patients may prove to be a liability in the rapidly approaching new healthcare system, as lack of engagement of the patient in the care relationship may result in less than optimal outcomes. Never has a strong relationship between provider and patient been needed as much as now.

Patients, along with their providers, must have a solid understanding of their health and how, as patients, they can influence their health status through behavior. Patients must be exposed to vital information that is used to drive the providers' diagnosis and treatment suggestions. Exposure to this data may be comforting, and understanding this information is empowering.

Truly informed decisions can occur only when complete transparency is present. One cannot make good decisions if material is not understood. Lack of knowledge, on the part of either the patient or the provider, opens the door to error. Decisions made using incomplete knowledge are not informed decisions. With clarity of understanding, patients are able to apply value to their options and truly weigh their decisions based on their own quality of life definition and their personal health goals.

Much like the aforementioned Dickens classic, healthcare is in a revolution. Present transitions in healthcare are moving toward a true patient-centered delivery system. Medagogy focuses on meeting the patient where they are in their health, in their knowledge, and in their goals. Health sustainability is contingent on responsible self-care. Patient education is the key to success in healthcare because it is the enabling factor that allows patients to assume their rightful position of control in their healthcare treatment.

For more information about Medagogy tools and courses please visit www.organizationofpatienteducators.com or email formedagogyinfo@gmail.com.

Expert Perspectives on Field Utilization and Implementation

Trenton L. James, MD, FAAFP, CPE
Baton Rouge Medical Center

Melissa Stewart's writings and teachings have brought definition to patient education—a complex and important part of treatment. She brings reason and know-how to all healthcare professionals, assisting their efforts in this most noble and essential part of patient care. Dr. Stewart helps the reader find and champion the teachable moment.

After years of practicing family medicine and offering one-on-one education to my patients, it is exciting to finally find evidence-based insights for what truly works along with tools that will improve this art of medicine. In the past, supporting patients who traveled from my care into the realm of self-care was often hit-or-miss. This book is a valuable guide for discovering how and when the patient is able to absorb the lessons that we know are critical to saving and improving the quality of their lives.

In our quest to achieve a longer life expectancy, we found that adding years to a patient's life also brings the danger of more time spent in costly chronic disease states. As we guard against this potential in a system struggling to change and reform, we must draft the patient as a partner. Our focus will shift to vigilant prevention and wellness care, early disease diagnosis, disease management, and care coordination; a knowledgeable patient is critical to the success of this transition in healthcare.

Patients with multiple complex problems, on multiple medications from multiple providers, must be educated (along with caregivers) to self-care and self-help. They also have a responsibility to fully engage with their providers. It will improve the quality of their healthcare and, in so doing, will improve their lives. This book will help the reader become a better-educated partner with their empowered patient.

Read this book, study it, and keep it close at hand. Your patients deserve it and quality outcomes demand it!

Michelle Jewell, RN, CPE
Administrator
Clarity Hospice

Just hearing the word "hospice" brings all sorts of emotions to the surface—death, dying, giving up, pain, loss of loved ones, regret, and probably the greatest emotion of all, FEAR. So as a healthcare provider, teaching a patient or family member the benefits of hospice can be extremely challenging. This is where being a certified patient educator (CPE) training on the Medagogy conceptual framework has provided me the greatest benefit.

Hospice service is one of the most effective and beneficial services that healthcare provides, yet it is sorely underutilized. Many healthcare providers have difficulty explaining hospice benefits to patients and their families because of the implied message of dying associated with the service. When the hospice referral should occur, qualified candidates for services and their families most often are in a physical and emotional crisis and many do not know their terminal status.

Going through the CPE course made me realize that to be a true patient advocate I first had to partner with patients. Partnering with patients in their care should always be a priority, but especially at pivotal points in healthcare such as life-or-death decisions. It was my job to find out *who* the patient really was, *where they were* at that point in their healthcare, and *how did they want to proceed*. To be an effective caregiver, I had to learn whether they understood why they were diagnosed as terminal and then what was the patient's perception of his or her health status, options, and hospice services.

Using the PITS model opened the door for me to breach the taboo subject of hospice care. Once the patient's protective defenses were down and the patient knew that I was on their side, only then would they allow me to share the benefits of hospice care with them. Considering the number of factors influencing patients, it is amazing they are ever able to absorb any information while they are in the healthcare system!

I felt that my success was achieved when the patient, usually with the family's input, could make their choice on how they would like to live until they died. Through the use of Medagogy principles I have been able to connect with patients and help them reach their healthcare aspirations. The reward of providing peace through knowledge for my patients and their families has been personally rewarding for me.

Johnetta McCray Russ, RNC, BSN, LNC, CPE, BCBC

It was heartbreaking to hear things such as: "The 'care' has gone out of healthcare;" "nurses can't nurse like they use to;" and "technology has taken nurses away from the bedside." But it was even more heart-tugging to confront the fact that my own passion for nursing was waning. One day it was all about patient care and patients first. Seemingly overnight, it became all about new and improved technology, advanced degrees, certifications, and Magnet designations.

What had happened to good old-fashioned bedside nursing where the nurse took the time, and had the time, to educate her patients thoroughly? What had happened to the prestige of being a bedside nurse? The nurses on our unit passionately loved being at the bedside, but times were changing and all too soon we became painfully aware that we needed to be more than just "Susie RN at the bedside." "Susie" needed something more than just "RN" after her name. Our colleagues were advancing, seeking master's degrees and obtaining certifications, so we needed to advance, too. We feared that we were becoming "nursing dinosaurs."

We were challenged to find a way to balance nursing the way we loved it with professionally advancing alongside our healthcare counterparts. Being a same-day surgery unit in a specialty hospital posed a huge hurdle to conquer. We didn't want to become certified in just anything, it had to have real meaning for us. What we *knew* was that positive patient outcomes were a direct result of effective patient education beforehand. A well-informed patient impacts the continuum of care. There were few certifications that even remotely captured the essence of what we did. Thus, any real clinical match continually eluded us. One day, however, we stumbled upon a certification in Patient Education. Education of patients is what we did and what we loved. We thought we had died and gone to heaven. Seven nurses from our unit attended the Patient Education course and sat for the certification exam. We all passed the exam and currently represent the first of what we hope will be many CPE (certified patient educators) nurses at our facility.

The information we gained has been invaluable to our daily practice. This is the first time in many years that we have been excited about nursing and the future of professional nursing. One of my fellow CPEs eloquently summed up what it means for us to have this certification. "The techniques I have learned from the patient education course have once again empowered me to positively impact my nursing practice. In the midst of later patient arrival times, decreased admit assessment times, technological advances such as computerized documentation, etc., the PITS model has taught me how to zero-in on what my specific patient needs to know. Sometimes I have more time than others to spend with a patient, but now *each* time I feel confident that I have met my patient where her educational need was and have given her what she needed before leaving my unit".

We are honored to be a part of this excellent opportunity to see patient education take its rightful place: impacting healthcare and putting the "care" back into *healthcare*. Patient literacy should be a top priority for every healthcare professional. As healthcare providers, we are patient advocates, and our patients need to be "in the know."

SECTION I

SHIFTING THE FOCUS TO THE PATIENT

[CHAPTER 1]

The Problem of Health Literacy

Health is an elusive concept for which there is no universal definition. Health has been defined as a state of well-being, optimal physical condition, and desired shape and strength. Much like beauty, health is in the eye of the beholder; personal interpretation impacts an individual's definition of health. Historically, the healthcare system has assumed authority in the acquisition of health. Through knowledge, expertise, and influence, healthcare providers attempt to assist people on their quest for health.

For years healthcare providers have discussed the notion of partnering with patients, the consumers of their services. Partnering brings a sense of equality and shared control to the relationship. Unfortunately, the varying levels of knowledge and differing perspectives among patients have been barriers to the partnership. This lack of shared understanding has impeded the provider and patient from merging their perceptions into a unified effort to achieve health.

Never has the need for provider-patient partnership been greater than now. As healthcare moves from a reactive delivery model to a proactive delivery model, the provider and patient must be in sync to achieve optimal health outcomes. A foundation of shared understanding can be built by improving patient education through establishing definition and structure. Cultivating patient knowledge through education must become a focus of the healthcare industry in order for preventive medicine and provider-patient partnership to occur.

Patient knowledge is the subject of interest for this book. The focus is on the information exchange process that occurs in the patient-provider

3

relationship in the healthcare system. The process of patient education is reviewed according to the medagogy model. The medagogy model works to identify information flow throughout the process of patient education. The concepts and relationships of medagogy serve as the core of a training program for Certified Patient Educators (CPE).

Today, healthcare is a focus of national concern. Rudimentary problems like inappropriate access with lack of fair and prudent resource utilization plague our present healthcare delivery model ("Access," 2005; Beyer, 2009; Bodenheimer & Fernandez, 2005; Evans, 2004; Ginsburg, 2004; Hanks, 1994; Lambrew, 2004; McLaughlin, 2008; Twanmoh & Cunningham, 2006; White, 1999). Proposed solutions to meeting the growing health needs of the nation and the world include greater access to providers and insurance coverage, and improved preventive services (Bailey, 1995; Esposito, Luchette, & Gamell, 2006; Lancaster et al., 2009; Thompson et al., 2009). Although these proposed solutions can help address present healthcare concerns, movement toward active patient involvement can help relieve the present dependency of patients that is exhausting our healthcare system (Prilleltensky, 2005). The public's dependency on the healthcare system has been linked to health literacy. For the healthcare delivery system to leave its current reactive delivery structure and move toward a new proactive delivery approach, massive systemic change must occur (Karpf, Lofgren, & Perman, 2009; Lofgen, Karpf, Perman, & Higdon, 2006; Whitehead, 2006).

Initially, healthcare providers need to look beyond the boundaries of their practice setting and the present moment in time into the future of health for each patient they see. Although the patient may present with an acute condition, preventive healthcare will require the provider to make a time-oriented change in treatment focus to include present care and prospective health needs. Health promotion and successful disease prevention lie in early intervention (Breslow, 1999; Maibach, Van Duyn, & Bloodgood, 2006). Point-of-service treatment will not be limited to the patient's past and present health, as historically seen in healthcare; it must also include action for patients' future health concerns. The individual's presenting health status, lifestyle, and family history are a few pieces of data that can help a provider identify future health risks. Providers will need to address and prepare the patient for future conditions that may threaten the patient's health. Through education providers can prepare patients for present and prospective health issues along with possible challenges that may be encountered in the future.

Case Study

John, the town's chief of police, is a 45-year-old African American male with high blood pressure, a family history of maternal and paternal heart disease, and a pack-a-day cigarette habit. He presents in the clinic for complaints of flu-like symptoms. Although flu-like symptoms are the reason that the patient accessed the system and are his immediate treatment need, his profile based on history and lifestyle habits provide an opportunity to establish proactive interventions for certain risks that may lead to future health problems. If the risks progress into actual diseases, the patient may lose more than his health status. The transition from risk to actual health problems can rob the patient of quality of life, independence, financial security, and even life itself. The providers' glimpse into the potential future for this patient's health warrants action. Treatment of the acute-state flu-like symptoms is the first priority because that is the patient's main concern, but investing in the patient's future health by empowering him with information may be life-saving.

Expert Support for Action

Cardiovascular disease research consistently references stabilizing acute conditions before initiating any preventive measures (McPhee et al., 2007; Raczynski & DiClemente, 1999). Falvo (2004) asserts that patient education focused on prevention is most effective if the patient's perceived needs and immediate concerns are first addressed.

Treatment

John is treated for his flu-like symptoms. First, Dr. Flowers, the internist, teaches John about what is causing his present symptoms, signs that his condition may be worsening, action to take if symptoms worsen, and how to carry out his ordered treatment plan. He then schedules a follow-up visit. Next, he tells John that his history and lifestyle put him at risk for cardiac disease and long-term complications. Dr. Flowers then establishes intent to focus on prospective cardiac issues on John's next visit. On John's follow-up visit, assessment reveals that John's initial health issue is resolved, so Dr. Flowers begins to expose John to information regarding his cardiac risk.

Ultimately, the provider of healthcare services will need to take past and present information from the patient's health history, clinical and laboratory findings, observed signs, and the patient's symptoms to render an expert opinion for present and future health needs.

Patients need to be as independent as possible regarding their healthcare, although there may be times when the patient regresses to a more dependent state, such as in the case of a severe acute myocardial infarction (AMI) (Falvo, 2004). In treatment of severe AMI, the patient is totally dependent on the healthcare provider; the only thing a patient can do in this case is follow direction and answer questions. Once the AMI is stabilized and the situation is under control, then the patient is more likely capable of assuming some self-care; simple activities of daily living like brushing teeth and combing hair are tasks that the patient may be able to resume.

When the patient is not in a critical health situation, the patient and the provider should partner to maximize opportunity for improved health status. Healthcare providers need to investigate beyond the physical assessment so that treatment can be tailored to meet the patient's individual health needs (Falvo, 2004; Redman, 2004). Values, goals, priorities, and idiosyncrasies that are specific to each individual will provide direction for health promotion, disease prevention, health resolution, and health maintenance. To meet the provider's informational needs, the patient will need to educate the provider about his condition, lifestyle, and personal habits that may impact health status. The patient's expertise about himself will help guide the provider and empower the patient to participate in the planning of his own individual care. Likewise, the provider, who serves as the healthcare expert in the patient-provider relationship, will need to educate the patient on the functions of his body, how disease impacts its functions, and how suggested treatment options can help address his health. Together, the two experts will forge a treatment plan oriented to the patient's life and the provider's understanding of applicable resources and patient ability.

The patient, as expert of self, bears responsibility in the patient-provider relationship to educate the provider on self and personal life situations; the provider is obligated to provide the patient with a full rationale for the suggested treatment plan. Possessing an understanding of why something should be done affords the patient the opportunity to prioritize this health information into his world. Redman (2004) recognizes the healthcare professional as the gatekeeper of healthcare knowledge. A patient's lack of exposure to professional healthcare rationale or knowledge limits the patient's power in managing his healthcare. Patient education empowers patients so they are able to influence the direction and course of their personal healthcare, thereby increasing their health autonomy.

A common ground of understanding can be achieved through active expert exchange of information in the patient-provider relationship. This common repository of information is called shared knowledge. The healthcare system is the milieu for patient care transitioning. The healthcare system must master the exchange of patient and treatment information between healthcare providers, entities, and systems. The informational hand-off between providers should include historical and present physical health status, treatment, and progression of patient knowledge. Exchange of patient knowledge can offer a foundation on which to build new information. Being aware of how well the patient understands his health status allows subsequent providers to build on the efforts that have been exerted to help educate the patient prior to the present point of care. Well documented in the literature is the fact that healthcare providers at various points of care either over- or underestimate both patients' understanding of their health and desire for information (Keulers, Schelting, Houterman, Van Der Wilt, & Spauwen, 2008; Schwartzberg, 2002).

In the ideal progression of the patient health knowledge delivery model, provider understanding of previous patient educational effort would allow new teaching efforts to refresh and expand on the prior work of other providers. Each provider would build on the patient's knowledge, allowing patients to move toward higher levels of comprehension and independence regarding their health and self-care. The system supports the provider's and patient's knowledge progression as they move toward a common domain of shared knowledge. Figure 1-1 displays the shared knowledge domain necessary for the provider and patient to create a healthcare plan in partnership.

Patient education is a basic yet vital element of healthcare that must be addressed to ensure successful outcomes (Smith, Dixon, Trevena, Nutbeam, & McCaffery, 2009). In the challenge of creating a new, divergent healthcare delivery system, patient education can facilitate our passage into a new paradigm of healthcare constructed around a provider-patient relationship where health goals and treatment choices are the products of mutually shared and gained understanding (Prilleltensky, 2005). *Shared knowledge* is defined as *general information universally understood by all parties.* Shared knowledge is identified in Figure 1-1 as the overlapping portions of individual circles that represent the patient, the provider, and the healthcare system. The knowledge shared among the patient, provider, and healthcare system serves as a foundation on which new knowledge can be

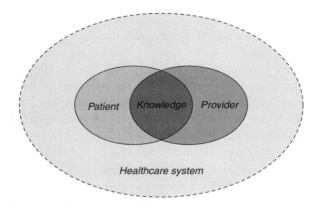

Figure 1-1. Shared knowledge domains. The domains of knowledge for patient, provider, and healthcare system are displayed. The provider and patient are both working within the healthcare system. The intersection of the provider, the patient, and the healthcare system depicts the common knowledge shared by all three domains.

constructed. Shared knowledge is also a connection between parties that can be used to gain a greater understanding about one another.

In the healthcare system, the shared domain of knowledge between experts—the provider and the patient—allocates assigned control and power to both parties in the partnership. Only the patient knows what he truly wants to gain from his healthcare. Therefore, patients need to maintain their right to manage their health by having control in their healthcare (Cagle & Kovacs, 2009). Patient education is a conduit to help patients assume their rightful collaborative role in the patient-provider relationship. Patient education has moved from a narrow medical illness–related approach of patient teaching to a broader paradigm of personal empowerment and participation, inclusive of health promotion, self-care, and disease prevention (Cagle & Kovacs, 2009; Roter, Satashesky-Margalit, & Rudd, 2001).

Health literacy is a term that used to communicate a level of proficiency and skill associated with healthcare and/or health maintenance. Presently, the term *health literacy* means the level of competency in health maintenance a patient possesses. The receiver of health services, the patient, is the focus of health literacy in today's healthcare setting. Because health literacy does not occur in a vacuum, lack of thorough understanding is an issue for both patient and provider, and health literacy problems are exacerbated as a patient cycles through the healthcare system desperately seeking a solution to their health needs. The maze of broken communication and inconsistency among providers in our reactive delivery system perpetuates confusion and compounds the unrealistic expectations placed on patients. Success in healthcare requires successful communication from both parties in the provider-patient partnership.

Identifying skills the patient lacks is only one aspect of addressing the patient's health literacy. The provider's knowledge-deficit of the patient's interpretation of health needs, patient values, and how behavioral changes fit into the patient's definition of quality of life leaves the provider with a patient literacy issue that must also be addressed. To better appreciate the need for an informed patient, the problem of health literacy needs to be examined in detail.

HEALTH LITERACY TODAY

To receive all that healthcare has to offer, health literacy skills are vital for the patient (Boswell, Cannon, Aung, & Eldridge, 2004; Tkacz, Metzgner, & Pruchnicki, 2008). *Health literacy* is defined by the United States Department of Health and Human Service, the National Library of Medicine, the Center for Health Care Strategies, and the Institute of Medicine (IOM) as the aptitude to gain, interpret, and utilize basic health information and understand what assistance is needed to make appropriate healthcare decisions (Center for Disease Control, 2007; Center for Health Strategies, Inc, 2005; Mancuso, 2008; US Department of Health and Human Services, 2008). The World Health Organization (WHO) includes patient motivation (Kickbusch, 2001), while the American Medical Association (AMA) adds the ability to measure and use numbers to their definition (Greenburg, 2001; Mancuso, 2008). Nutbeam (2000) inserts personal-life context into his health literacy definition, which adds individual situation and priorities to the individual's health status. Health literacy has various meanings and definitions with no common construct, making health literacy a challenge to measure and fully study (Baker, 2006). Healthy People 2010 includes goals to improve the health literacy crisis (Centers for Disease Control, 2007). Healthy People 2020 retained Healthy People 2010's health literacy objectives and moved them under the heading of health communication/health information technology initiatives (Secretary's Advisory Committee on National Health Promotion and Disease Prevention, 2009).

The following definition takes into account skills needed from all involved in healthcare: *health literacy is the level of health understanding, inclusive of personal values and priorities, which frames health decisions and results in health action through behavior change determined from individual interpretation.* Providers and patients both use their values and knowledge to make healthcare decisions. Actions resulting from decisions are determined from personal meaning. Health choices can impact quality of life. Behavior change resulting from healthcare choices may range from extreme to no action. Whatever action is chosen, the choice lies with the individual since quality of life is individually defined. If the requested action is not viewed as a priority by one party, then a struggle of goals between provider and patient will occur. Mutual health goals established through acceptance of each other's values and choices can deliver achievable health outcomes.

HISTORY OF HEALTH LITERACY

Health literacy has been a catchphrase since it was first uttered in 1974 (Simonds, 1978), and is a colossal problem in healthcare in the United States and around the world (Betz, Ruccione, Meeske, Smith, & Chang, 2008; Carter & Wallace, 2007). In the 1990s, the field of health literacy became a trendy focus for research in response to society's sobering new awareness of the strong association between health and education (White, 2008). In 1998, seven statements were incorporated into the Patient's Bill of Rights that addressed information patients receive and acknowledged a patient's right to know about health status, care options, and requirements for care (U.S. Department of Health and Human Services, 1999). Osborne (2005), a health literacy expert, acknowledges the importance of literacy by heightening awareness that life-threatening mistakes happen when patients cannot read or comprehend health information. Even well-educated Americans have difficulty understanding medical jargon, medical forms, and prescription information (Burnham & Peterson, 2005; Committee on Health Literacy, 2004). Barrett and Puryear (2006) state that all patients, from the well educated to those with limited literacy skills, are vulnerable to misunderstanding, not comprehending, and being unable to act on directions from healthcare providers. Clear, patient-oriented provider communication increases understanding and decreases confusion in the patient population (Barrett & Puryear, 2006; Sudore & Schillinger, 2009).

INTERNATIONAL HEALTH LITERACY

Health illiteracy is not endemic to the United States, and is crossing borders throughout the world. Switzerland, Australia, New Zealand, and other countries are also struggling with the challenge of health literacy (Stableford & Mettger, 2007). Canadian and European patients may have easier access to healthcare through their nationalized healthcare systems, but these regions also fight health illiteracy as their healthcare consumers struggle to read, understand, and use information essential to preventing, treating, and properly managing complex health conditions. The World Health Organization and the European Commission reports highlight that effective communication is critical to public understanding of health information (Stableford & Mettger, 2007). The American Institute of Medicine, Agency for Healthcare Research, and Health Association Libraries Section, a section of the Medical Library Association, all have produced reports that stress the same need that the World Health Organization (WHO) and the European Commission's reports request: a need for clear, congruent, legitimate information (Stableford & Mettger, 2007) that is relevant and culturally competent.

The Canadian Public Health Association (CPHA) claims that low health literacy is a serious and costly problem that will become worse as the Canadian population ages and the incidence of chronic disease proliferates (Canadian Public Health Association, 2008). The CPHA proposes that improving health literacy will lead to decreased healthcare costs and improved outcomes. Enhanced communication can improve health literacy and can ultimately reduce a nation's overall healthcare burden by decreasing dependency on healthcare by empowering people with health skills (Furnee, Groot, & Maassen van den Brink, 2008; Monachos, 2007).

The Institute of Medicine (IOM) and the Agency for Healthcare Research and Quality (AHRQ), two major agencies in the United States healthcare system, both issued health literacy reports in 2004 that placed the topic of health literacy at the forefront of the nation's health agenda (Stableford & Mettger, 2007). The WHO's 6th Global Conference acknowledged that health-promoting strategies provide equal learning opportunities for all people to achieve basic health literacy and are an essential duty for all levels of government (Stableford & Mettger, 2007). The WHO report notes that clear, uninhibited communication is a critical for effective promotion of health (Stableford & Mettger, 2007). Effective healthcare-provider communication strategies are essential to mobilize individuals toward healthy options and increase the likelihood of choices that could produce healthy behaviors (Stableford & Mettger, 2007).

PREVALENCE OF HEALTH LITERACY

Unlike a broken arm, an abnormal blood pressure, or even an elevated blood glucose level, there are no physical signs or symptoms that alert a healthcare provider to a silent, costly, and crippling health problem: a lack of essential health literacy skills. There is no age, no race, no sex, no face, and there is little to no social differentiation between a person who is health literate and one who has poor health literacy. Though found in all segments of society, Americans born and raised in the United States represent the majority of the population with poor health literacy (Weiss, 2007). Poor health literacy in the United States is characterized as public health's "silent epidemic" (Marcus, 2006). The percentage of people with insufficient health literacy skills has increased from 40% of the United States' adult population in 1992 to greater than 50% in 2004, or approximately 90 million people (Maniaci, Heckman, & Dawson, 2008). The 2003 National Healthcare Disparities Report from the National Assessment of Adult Health Literacy found that 12% of Americans have proficient health literacy skills, 53% have intermediate skills, and 36% have basic to low health literacy skills (AHRQ, 2006; Health literacy in the United States, 2008). Maniaci, Heckman, and Dawson (2008) state that advances in healthcare technology and complications of healthcare delivery have made it more difficult to assess a patient's ability to understand complex medical information.

IMPACT OF EDUCATION ON HEALTH LITERACY IN THE UNITED STATES

Evidence supports a positive relationship between education and health (Furnee et al., 2008). According to the United States Department of Labor, 47% of the adult population of the United States has poor literacy and 10% to 14% of adults in the workforce have a learning disability. One out of every five patients is functionally literate (Kirsch, Jungeblut, Jenkins, & Kolstad, 2002). A study of 445 adult female subjects with fourth grade literacy skills found that 39% did not understand why women get mammograms (Davis et al., 1998). A study of 3,260 elderly subjects found a relationship between educational attainment and health status (Howard, Sentell, & Gazmararian, 2006).

Literacy level is not always reflective of educational level, but is strongly associated with employment, community membership, and health status (Health Canada, 1999). A 2002 study that reviewed claims for a Medicare managed-care company for two years found that low-literate enrollees had a 52% higher risk of hospital admission (Baker et al., 2002). Seventy-five percent of chronically ill American adults possess low literacy skills (Cutilli & Bennett, 2009; Prasauskas & Spoo, 2006).

Most health education is written at a high school level, although the average Medicaid recipient reads at only a fifth grade level (U.S. Department of Labor, 2001). The average Medicare recipient reads at a sixth grade level (GAO, 2006). To add to the complexity, healthcare has its own vernacular that is unfamiliar to most people. Patient education products often burden the reader with complex medical verbiage that confuses the reader (Schwartzenburg, Corrett, Vangeest, 2005). A 1997 study discovered that even college-educated individuals have difficulty interpreting and using medical information (Schwartz, Woloshin, Black, & Welch, 1997).

Many patients hide their misunderstandings and literacy limitations because of shame or embarrassment (Kripalani & Weiss, 2006). Most healthcare professionals are not trained to help patients deal with their feelings of shame related to literacy (Schwartzenberg, Corrett, VanGeest, & Wolf, 2007). Patients often do not admit that they do not know. Some patients feel inept and incapable of asking their healthcare physician questions (Leydon et al., 2000; McKenzie, 2000).

ETHNIC AND ELDER DISPARITY

Poor health literacy has been found to be more common in ethnic minorities and the elderly (Committee on Understanding and Eliminating Racial and Ethnic Disparities in Health Care, 2003; Schillinger et al., 2002). One study found that 42% of 202 African-Americans surveyed acknowledged inadequate health literacy (Parikh, Parker, Nurss, Baker, & Williams, 1996). The growth in poor health literacy is rapidly outpacing advances in healthcare technology; therefore, to meet patients' basic needs to understand, healthcare providers must concentrate their efforts on addressing the problem of health literacy through scientific exploration of potential solutions (Greenburg, 2001; Raynor, 2008; Sorrell, 2006). Low health literacy presents challenges to medication identification (Kripalani et al.,

2006) and to medication self-management (Davis & Wolf, 2006; Kripalani et al., 2006; Wolf et al., 2007). A study of 85 subjects with low literacy levels showed that they found medication labels confusing and difficult to understand (Webb et al., 2008). Another study found that by addressing medication misunderstandings, clinicians create a foundation on which to build new knowledge so patients can be more self-sufficient in their care (Spiers, Kutzik, & Lamar, 2004).

HEALTH LITERACY'S FINANCIAL IMPACT

Health spending in the United States is expected to top the overall national market increase by 3% per year, resulting in a growth from 13% of gross domestic product (GDP) in 2009 to 17% in 2010 (Gross Domestic Report: Third quarter 2009, 2009; National Health Expenditure Data, 2010). The Center for Medicare and Medicaid Services (CMS) predicts that by 2019 health spending in the United States will be $4.5 trillion (Pickert, 2010). Low health literacy inflicts a heavy financial impact on the overall cost of healthcare. The report entitled *Health Literacy: A Prescription to End Confusion,* released by the Institute of Medicine, estimated that the health literacy problem generates an annual cost of $73 billion (Committee on Health Literacy, 2004). In 2007, the estimated annual price tag of low health literacy increased to between $106 and $236 billion (Vernon, Trujillo, Rosenbaum, and DeBuono, 2007). These funds are spent because patients do not understand the communications and expectations of their health providers (Roberts, 2004).

The costs and utilization of healthcare services tracked through claims files of the participants revealed that enrollees with inadequate health literacy skills incurred higher medical costs than enrollees with adequate health literacy skills (Howard, Ganzmararian, & Parker, 2005). The Short Test of Functional Health Literacy was used to measure the health literacy of 3,260 participants, revealing that 800 subjects had inadequate health literacy skills, 366 subjects had marginal health literacy skills, and 2,094 subjects had adequate health literacy skills. The cost and utilization of healthcare services were then tracked through the participants' claims files. The data revealed that subjects with inadequate health literacy skills incurred higher medical costs when compared to enrollees with adequate health literacy skills (Howard et al., 2005). Individuals with limited health literacy skills have difficulty understanding their medication labels, suffer increased risk of hospitalization related to misunderstanding about self-care, and utilize fewer preventive services (Harper, 2007).

People with poor health literacy or diminished health understanding are directly impacted because they experience less than optimal health outcomes (Schwartzberg, 2002). The lack of understanding about how to take medicine correctly or read food labels to maintain dietary restrictions are two examples of common health literacy errors. Everyone is affected by the financial impact caused by inappropriate use and access of the healthcare system, increased length of stay (Weiss et al., 1994), extra healthcare provider visits (Harper, 2007), and recidivism (Baker et al., 2002; Weiss et al., 1994).

Though copious data helps to identify the problem and its ravenous consumption of healthcare resources, low health literacy remains a major issue. A lack of patient understanding leads to return visits, recidivism, increased financial burden, and less than optimal health outcomes (Harper, 2007). Healthcare reform offers an opportunity for patient education to become a central priority in healthcare. Improving health literacy can decrease a nation's overall healthcare costs (Furnee et al., 2008; Monachos, 2007).

As the cost of healthcare continues to surge, there is a growing acknowledgement that consumers must become active participants in their own healthcare. Healthcare reform is a monumental paradigm shift that aims to transition our nation's healthcare from a reactive delivery system to a patient-centered, proactive, preventive, and predictive model. To achieve a healthcare environment where consumers and providers both participate in treatment decision making, patients must have a better understanding of their health status and providers must have a good understanding of the patient's perspective and self-efficacy to adhere to a treatment regimen (Boswell, Cannon, Aung, & Eldridge, 2004; Tkacz, Metzgner, & Pruchnicki, 2008).

Recognizing the need for the provider to learn from the patient is a major challenge that may aid in resolving the issue of poor health literacy. It is crucial for the provider to learn from the patient, to understand the patient's perspective, and act upon patient-communicated information. Personal information from the patient can assist the provider in the formulation of a truly individualized plan of care (Redman, 2004). Information shared between the patient and provider forms the foundation of understanding from which both parties draw healthcare conclusions. The provider develops treatment options from information received from the patient. The patient creates personal relevance from the information received from the provider. There must be congruence and a sense of mutual trust between the two individuals for effective communication to occur.

SUMMARY

- Much like beauty, health is in the eye of the beholder; personal interpretation impacts an individual's definition of health.

- Never has the need for provider-patient partnership been more crucial than now. As healthcare moves from a reactive delivery model to a proactive delivery model, the provider and patient must be in sync to achieve optimal health outcomes.

- The process of patient education will be reviewed according to the medagogy model throughout this book. The medagogy model works to identify information flow throughout the process of patient education.

- When the patient is not in a critical health situation, the patient and provider should partner to maximize opportunity for improved health status.

- Through active expert exchange of information in the patient-provider relationship, a common ground of understanding can be achieved. This common understanding is called shared knowledge.

- Well documented in the literature is the fact that healthcare providers at various points of care either over- or underestimate patients' understanding of their health and desire for information.

- In the healthcare system, the shared domain of knowledge between experts—the provider and the patient—allocates assigned control and power to both parties in the partnership.

- Health literacy is the level of health understanding, inclusive of personal values and priorities, which frames health decisions and results in health action through behavior change determined from individual interpretation. Both the provider and patient use their values and knowledge to make healthcare decisions.

- Clear, patient-oriented provider communication offers an opportunity to increase understanding and decrease confusion in the patient population.

- The National Healthcare Disparities Report from the National Assessment of Adult Health Literacy found in its 2003 survey that 12% of Americans have proficient health literacy skills to manage their healthcare, 53% have intermediate skills, and 36% have basic to low health literacy skills. Recognizing the need for the provider to learn from the patient is a major challenge for resolving the issue of poor health literacy.

CHAPTER 2

The Patient's Perspective

Health literacy needs to shift from a disease-oriented approach to a patient-oriented one. In fact, the term *health literacy* should be replaced with the term *patient literacy*. The focus should be on formulating information specific to each patient; educators must be sure to consider who, where, and how the patient is at a particular point in time or season of health. Every patient needs education, and it is crucial to plan and deliver the necessary information based on each person's physical and psychological situation at that moment in time.

 ## Case Study

Jamie is a new mother. Like all new mothers Jamie needs to understand how to change a baby's diaper. But Jamie has experience changing babies' diapers. She works in the daycare by the hospital and she lives next door to her sister who has three small children. Including Jamie's experience when evaluating her patient education needs may help a healthcare team focus on knowledge-needs that are more appropriate. Compared with other first-time mothers, Jamie may not require as much information regarding diaper changing.

Expert Support for Action

Patient education is a legal responsibility of every licensed healthcare provider (Kraut, 1981). The Joint Commission requires accredited health institutions to identify and address each patient's health knowledge needs and encourages healthcare providers to partner with patients through information exchange and active patient participation in planning and execution of healthcare (The Joint Commission [TJC], 2007). The more that is known about the person the more the information can be personalized (Boothman, 2002). To have constructive dialogue, a platform of shared knowledge is required between provider and patient (Makoul, 2003). Providers need to gain an understanding of the patient from the information they receive from their patients (Hahn, 2009; Weiner, Barnet, Chang, & Daaleman, 2005).

 ## Case Study

Ashley, an eight-year-old girl with asthma, is quite proficient with the use of her inhaler. Ashley has suffered with asthma since the age of five. Over the years Ashley has not only mastered using her inhaler but also knows how to identify when her body is telling her she needs to use it. Ashley has become so comfortable with her inhaler skill that she helped her neighbor Joe, a 30 year old newly diagnosed with asthma, when he could not figure out how to activate his inhaler. It is important to note that age and skill cannot always be correlated.

Expert Support for Action

Through knowledge, a patient can cope with poor health and altered health states, potentially improving health outcomes and enhancing quality of life (Cooper et al., 2001). There is no age, no race, no sex, no face, and there is little to no social differentiation between a person who is health literate and one who has poor health literacy (Stewart, 2009).

There is a need to transition patient education from a global, standardized, one-size-fits-all model to an individually focused effort tailored specifically for each person. Maniaci and colleagues (2008) affirm that adequate patient-centered communication is needed to improve patient understanding. Patients must adequately understand their medical circumstances to interact effectively with their healthcare providers and to actively participate in the healing process (Maniaci, Heckman, & Dawson, 2008). Maniaci and colleagues (2008) assert that patients' abilities to understand can impact their independence, safety, cost of care, and overall health outcomes.

Health literacy is constantly being redefined, and it is crucial to resolve the issues of patients not understanding their health status or their providers' recommendations, which result in patients' dependence on the healthcare system (Centers for Disease Control, 2007; Center for Health Strategies, Inc, 2005; Mancuso, 2008; U.S. Department of Health and Human Services, 2008). In an attempt to address health literacy, Edmunds (2005) proposes that all health material for the general population be written and communicated at fifth- to seventh-grade levels to improve the odds of patients understanding the content. Empirical literature substantiates the opposite position—that limited universal levels are not effective for all patients (Billek-Sawhney & Reicherter, 2005; Hoffman & McKenna, 2006; Kripalani et al., 2001; Kripalani et al., 2006).

Mayer advocates for providers to meet the individual patient at their level of need (Roberts, 2004), which would require educator training for healthcare providers in assessment skills of patients' learning needs and information delivery. Because people have varying learning styles and different literacy levels, patient education needs to be designed to accommodate each individual's educational capabilities (Kurashige, 2008). Studies show that individualized instructions increase comprehension and memory more effectively than standardized instructions (Morrow et al., 2005; Robinson et al., 2008). Healthcare providers need to present information in a manner each patient can understand, recall, and use in their life and in making healthcare choices (Stableford & Mettger, 2007).

Empirical data identifying the seriousness of the health literacy crisis have prompted an appeal for trained healthcare providers to effectively educate patients (Kripalani et al., 2008; Schillinger et al., 2002; Visser, Deccache, & Bensing, 2001). Baker and colleagues assert that "it may be beneficial to think of limited health literacy analogously to physical disabilities: wheelchair-bound patients are not expected to climb stairs to access healthcare" (Baker et al., 2002, p. 1283). Similar to the accommodations that are mandated for patients with disabilities, "health care information should be made available to all patients regardless of their reading ability" (Baker et al., 2002, p. 1283).

It is assumed that if a healthcare provider knows a patient's literacy level, he or she can make adjustments to ensure that the information the patient receives will match the patient's literacy level (Greenburg, 2001). A study of 182 diabetic patients and 63 physicians revealed that physicians did not feel they possessed the skills needed to adequately adapt information to each patient's educational needs (Seligman et al., 2005). Most healthcare providers do not know how to adjust information or engage in patient teaching using educational principles and theories. A meta-analysis reviewed multiple types of patient educational interventions and found that theoretical models and educational frameworks were absent (Cooper, Booth, Fear, & Gill, 2001). Educational theory is necessary to guide patient teaching (Glanz, Rimer, & Viswanath, 2008). Personalized and theoretically grounded patient education is important to resolve the health literacy problem (Committee on Health Literacy, 2004).

Controversy exists regarding whether healthcare providers receive adequate training to be good patient educators (Chang & Kelly, 2007; Luker & Caress, 1988). While healthcare providers may be a valuable source of information, more training may be needed to allow them to be truly effective in patient education (Luker & Caress, 1988).

PATIENT EDUCATION

Skillful patient education can empower patients with health knowledge and control (Falvo, 1994; Redman, 2006). Healthcare providers often ad-lib the educational segments of their services to patients and fail to assign appropriate importance to this responsibility. This is unfortunate because patients rely on the knowledge and information gained from their providers to independently manage their healthcare needs (Kripalani & Weiss, 2006; Makoul, 2003). Unlike many other skills applied in healthcare, there is no global definition for patient education (Makoul, 2003). The National League of Nursing (NLN), in their 1976 publication *Patient Education*, defined patient education as the process of providing patients with knowledge, skill, competence, or desirable qualities of behavior. Phillips (1999) points out that patient teaching is the activity that is done to facilitate patient learning. Redman (2006) distinguishes patient education as a process of influence and planned learning. Redman states that in the patient education experience a combination of methods and techniques are used to influence patient knowledge and behavior (Redman, 2006). Patient education is also defined as "all educational activities, directed to patients, including aspects of therapeutic education, health education, and clinical health promotion" (Deccache & Aujoulat, 2001, p. 8). Patient education is "the process of assisting consumers of health care to learn how to incorporate health-related behaviors into everyday life for the purpose of achieving optimal health" (Bastable, 2006, p. 466).

For the purpose of this book, *patient education is defined as the act of purposeful patient engagement in activities that can impact a patient's knowledge through personal learning for future utilization, health autonomy, and long-term retention.* Patient learning includes the individual and personal processes of mental ingestion and absorption of information—planned and unplanned.

Brief Reflections on Patient Education History

In the eighteenth and nineteenth centuries, verbal communication and observation were the main sources of information for patient diagnosis and treatment (Reiser, 1981). Through the years, technology has threatened the relationship between patient and provider, distancing relationships and stifling verbal exchange. Nursing's participation in the practice of patient education is noted in the literature as far back as 1900 in the first volume, first edition of *American Journal of Nursing,* in the article "Visiting Nursing" authored by Eliza J. Moore. According to Falvo (1994), actual documentation of patient education within patient charts only dates back to the early 1950s. In the 1960s, the civil rights movement helped thrust social equality and empowerment into all areas, including healthcare (Rosen, 1977). During this same period, the American Medical Association (AMA) established an ethical commitment to patient education. In the seventies, the focus shifted to increasing awareness of patient education and patient rights, especially with the 1971 publication of *The Need for Patient Education* by the Department of Health, Education, and Welfare (Falvo, 1994). In 1973, the American Hospital Association (AHA) developed the *Patient's Bill of Rights* (American Hospital Association [AHA], 1973). Also in 1973, the American Nurses Association (ANA) published *ANA's Standards of Nursing Practice*, which identified nurses' responsibilities in patient education. The patient's bill of rights became regarded as an ethical guide to the delivery of healthcare through honoring patients' rights to information, involvement, and choice (NLN, 1976).

In 1975, the ANA published *The Professional Nurse and Health Education*, which delineated patient education as a responsibility of the

Registered Nurse from illness to health maintenance (ANA, 2004; Falvo, 1994). The 1975 ANA publication also indicated accountability on the part of the nurse, patient, and family for delivery of relevant appropriate information throughout the healthcare process (ANA, 1975). In 1980, the AMA sanctioned a new version of *Principles of Medical Ethics*, calling for physicians to make healthcare information available to patients. The Patient Self-Determination Act was enacted in December 1991. The Act enabled patients to make choices about end-of-life issues such as life support and other life-sustaining interventions through advanced directives (Markus, 1997). In March of 1998, the Patient's Bill of Rights became law (U.S. Department of Health and Human Services, 1999). All licensed healthcare providers were required to educate patients as outlined in seven statements in the Patient's Bill of Rights.

The focus of health literacy should deal with information that the patient receives while acknowledging the patient's right to know about personal health problems, health status, treatments, alternative care options, and continuing care requirements (U.S. Department of Health and Human Services, 1999). Figure 2-1 displays a historical timeline for health literacy education.

Although patient education has been part of the Joint Commission's standards since 1976 (Joint Commission on Accreditation of Healthcare Organizations, 1976), in March of 2002 the Center for Medicare and Medicaid Services (CMS), in partnership with the Joint Commission, launched a national public campaign called "Speak Up". The campaign was designed as a patient safety initiative to help prevent medical errors and healthcare mistakes by urging the lay population to get involved in their healthcare by asking questions and actively participating in their healthcare planning (The Joint Commission [TJC], 2010).

In February 2007, to help health professionals understand the impact health literacy was having on patient health and safety, the Joint Commission released the white paper, *"What Did the Doctor Say?": Improving Health Literacy to Protect Patient Safety.* The white paper highlighted the need for healthcare organizations to establish a safe patient environment across the care continuum through effective communication (The Joint Commission [TJC], 2007). The Joint Commission requires accredited health institutions to identify and address each patient's health-knowledge needs and encourages healthcare providers to partner with patients through information exchange and active patient participation in planning and execution of healthcare.

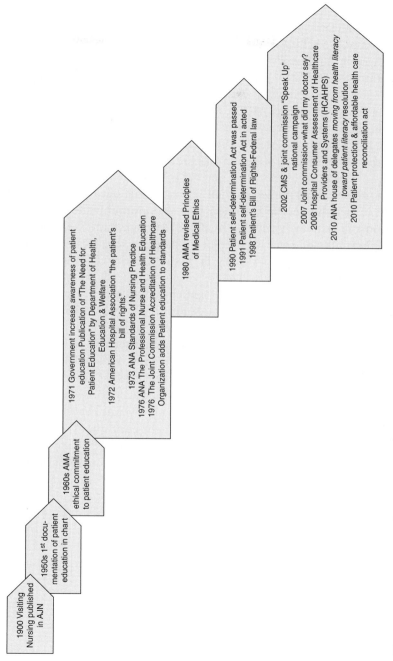

Figure 2-1. Historical timeline of events that are significant to patient education (CMS, 2011; Trossman, 2010; Falvo, 2004; Moore, 1900; Redman, 2004).

In 2008, some hospitals began voluntarily reporting Hospital Consumer Assessment of Healthcare Providers and Systems (HCACPS) results (CMS, 2011). In June 2010 the ANA's House of Delegates passed the resolution "Moving from health literacy toward patient literacy," making health literacy a major initiative for ANA (Trossman, 2010). Also in 2010, the Patient Protection and Affordability Act was signed into law. The Patient Protection and Affordability Act utilizes HCACPS as a measure to calculate provider payment in the Hospital Value-Based Purchasing Program effective in 2012 (CMS, 2011). Communication with the patient is reflected in HCACPS allowing the patient's interpretation of care to determine provider reimbursement.

Today, even with all the technologic advances that have been achieved– especially in healthcare–the common task of communication of health information still remains virtually undefined. Though patient education is a legal responsibility of every licensed healthcare provider (Kraut, 1981), it remains an unstructured and usually ill-planned exchange that occurs in patient-provider interactions (Clark & Gong, 2000; Clark, et al., 1997; Makoul, 2003). This lack of focus on patient education has perpetuated the previously discussed phenomenon of health illiteracy, which has had devastating effects on human health across the globe.

Literature reveals that patients want more information from their healthcare providers (Boberg et al., 2003; Jenkins, Fallowfield, & Saul, 2001). Providing patient information is a crucial part of clinical practice and directly influences a patient's satisfaction, compliance, self-management, independence, understanding, and overall health outcomes (Falvo, 2004; Redman, 2004). The goal of patient education is to increase the patients' knowledge and understanding of their health. Patient teaching can only be effective if the patient learns through meaningful dialogue and understands the information provided (Sorrell, 2006). Deficits in the distribution of patient information could be related to the provider underestimating the patient's needs and misjudging the patient's level of satisfaction with the information offered (Makoul, Arnston, & Schofield, 1995). Replacing providers' assumptions with good educational skills can empower patients with the knowledge and understanding needed to meet their health goals.

Ethics of Patient Education

Bioethics champions the patient's right to choice through informed consent (Knapp, 2006). Sullivan (2003) states that bioethics shifts the focus of healthcare toward patient-centeredness and challenges providers to expand their area of concern beyond patients' physical bodies to patients' lives and values. Patient education falls under the umbrella of bioethics, although it is addressed only peripherally through the doctrine of informed consent (Falvo, 2004).

Withholding or distorting patient information can be considered unethical and dangerous because it may lead to patient harm (Fallowfield & Jenkins, 1999; Redman, 2008). Falvo (2004) identifies the ethical responsibility that healthcare providers have to deliver information to patients in a fair, honest, and unbiased manner. Breach of this duty is noted in a paternalistic approach to healthcare delivery where providers assume control in the patient-provider relationship and use "because-I-said-so" reasoning with their patients. Limiting the information a patient receives can cultivate patient dependency on healthcare providers, which can lead to personal gain for some healthcare providers (Falvo, 2004).

Changes in Healthcare: Impact on Patient Education

Although the clinical encounter can still be very informative for healthcare providers, due to twentieth-century advances in biomedical technology the main sources of patient health information are retrieved from lab tests and machines versus verbal exchange with the patient (Roter, Satashefsky-Margalit, & Rudd, 2001). Roter and colleagues (2001) maintain that patient education has moved from a narrow illness–related approach to patient education toward a broader paradigm of personal empowerment and disease prevention. Studies focused on patient education for preventive health behaviors suggest that patient education positively contributes to disease prevention (Mullen et al., 1997). Studies have shown that patient education can increase patient knowledge (Devine, 2003; Glasson et al., 2006; Guevara et al., 2003). Patient safety (Lorenzen, Melby, & Earles, 2008; Ratzan, 2007) and health outcomes improve with progression of patients' health knowledge (Devine, 2003; Glasson et al., 2006; Guevara, Wolf, Grum, & Clark, 2003). Although this new paradigm is a sign that healthcare is moving in the right direction, patient education remains an ill-defined yet mandated licensed healthcare provider responsibility. To enable constructive dialogue, a platform of shared knowledge is required between provider and patient (Makoul, 2003).

Literature reveals that the health-knowledge needs of patients are not valued as much as their physical needs (Friberg, Bergh, & Lepp, 2006). Most licensed healthcare providers are not reimbursed for patient education (Miller, Hill, Ottke, & Ockene, 1997). This lack of reimbursement affects the allocation of resources and attention that are needed to make a significant impact in the health education of patients (Wagner et al., 2001). A lack of fiscal remuneration for patient education could be seen as an unspoken statement about the worth of patient education, implying that it is not a valuable duty in the hierarchy of healthcare.

THE NEED TO ACT

People are living longer, they are living sicker, and they are living sicker longer (Cromie, 2006; DeGregori, 2003). Research shows that more than 100 million residents of the United States (30% to 40% of the population) have one or more chronic diseases, and of that group, more than half are not receiving the appropriate care (Glasgow, Funnell, Bonomi, Beckham, & Wagner, 2002). Two-thirds of the Medicare population has more than four chronic illnesses (Wagner, 2004). In 2003, more than 95% of all Medicare expenditures were spent on the treatment of chronic illnesses like diabetes, congestive heart failure, and chronic obstructive pulmonary disease (Wagner, 2004). Chronic illnesses caused 40 million sick days, which resulted in more than $1 billion lost in productivity (Wagner, 2004). The alarming increase in the number of individuals with chronic illnesses, along with the increase in life expectancy, will place even more challenges on our already overtaxed healthcare system (Glasgow et al., 2002). A shift toward increasing the autonomy of healthcare consumers could provide needed relief for our overburdened healthcare system.

People may be living longer, but they do not feel any better; patient education is something that "can make life better for people" (Tattersall, 1995, p. 375). Personal adaptation and psychological adjustment are paramount for a chronically ill patient (Cooper et al., 2001). Through knowledge, a patient can cope with poor health and altered health states, improving health outcomes and enhancing quality of life (Cooper et al., 2001). Providers make treatment decisions with the goal of improving patients' health and lives, but quality of life should be defined individually and determined by the patient (Tattersall, 1995). Personal definitions of quality of life are seen every day in patients' actions of protest. Patients protest to assert their definition of quality of life as the basis for managing their health status. Refusing treatment or not participating in a therapeutic treatment regimen may be seen as a patient's assertion of his definition of quality of life. For example, a diabetic patient detouring from the treatment course by choosing to consume a piece of pie or cake regularly may be asserting his definition and views about quality of life. In many instances, such individuals are fully aware of the damage that will ensue.

 ## Case Study

Nana is the oldest living person in our little town. Nana is an Asian American female who is 102 years old. She lives at the nursing home in town. Nana ambulates with a walker and is able to assist with her activities of daily living. She has been living with diabetes mellitus since she was 42 years old. Nana has a history of hypertension, hyperlipidemia, peripheral vascular disease, and depression. At the age of 50, Nana had a total hysterectomy because she was diagnosed with and treated for cervical cancer. Nana also has osteoporosis and has developed a pronounced curvature in her spine. Nana ingests 14 different oral medications and has 2 injections administered daily. At the age of 71 Nana had a stroke that left her with residual right-sided weakness and poor vision. Since that time Nana has required 24-hour-a-day nursing assistance and has been a resident of Willow Woods Long-term Care Facility for 30 years. The estimated cost of caring for and maintaining Nana's health since her first diagnosed chronic illness is around $4 to $4.5 million. Willow Woods is proud of their famous resident Nana, the town's only Centenarian.

Expert Support for Action

Health spending in the United States is expected to top the overall national market increase by 3% per year, resulting in a growth from 13% of gross domestic product (GDP) in 2009 to 17% in 2010 (Gross Domestic Report: Third quarter 2009, 2009; National Health Expenditure Data, 2010). In 2007, the estimated annual price tag of low health literacy increased to between $106 and $236 billion (Vernon, Trujillo, Rosenbaum, & DeBuono, 2007). These funds are spent because patients do not understand the communications and expectations of their healthcare providers (Roberts, 2004).

PROVIDERS NEED TO KNOW HOW TO TEACH

Parker, Ratzan, and Lurie (2003) call for someone to take on the responsibility of educating the patient and for payers to reimburse patient educators for their educational services. Many Americans with the greatest healthcare needs, including the elderly, have the least capacity to understand and independently act upon the healthcare information that has been provided for them (Bayliss, Ellis, & Steiner, 2007). Healthcare providers' methods of communication often do not facilitate the patient's ability to receive, process, and utilize health information (Miller et al., 1997; Vernon et al., 2007).

A study of 182 patients with diabetes and 63 primary care physicians found that physicians did not feel they possessed the skills needed to adequately adjust information for each patient's educational needs (Seligman et al., 2005). To help providers learn how to deliver health information, the AMA's Ad Hoc Committee on Health Literacy proposed the inclusion of health literacy education in the training of healthcare providers (American Medical Association Ad Hoc Committee on Health Literacy for the Council on Scientific Affairs, 1999). A 2007 study published in the *American Journal of Healthy Behavior* reviewed the utilization standardized patients in the training of medical residents in patient education or patient-provider communication. The study found the utilization of standardized patients in patient education training to be an effective teaching technique for healthcare providers (Manning & Kripalani, 2007). Harper, Cook, and Makoul (2007) advocate for a task-oriented approach to teaching healthcare providers how to accommodate for health literacy; this approach would simply outline the task to be completed, e.g. "use plain language" and "check for understanding" (Harper, Cook, & Makoul, 2007). Good patient education serves as a foundation for quality care (Tattersall, 1995). Patient education may cost more in advance, but ultimately the cost of care will be less and money will be saved (Tattersall, 1995). Patient education can increase medical advice adherence, improve self-management of chronic disease, and increase the likelihood of better health outcomes (Billek-Sawhney & Reicherter, 2005).

PATIENT EDUCATION METHODS

There are a myriad of methods used for patient education in clinical practice. The most common methods are one-on-one instruction, lecture, demonstration, handouts or instructional booklets, and videos. Pictographs, which are pictures that health care professionals can use in the education of patients, are also helpful in relaying information (Greenburg, 2001). In a 1998 study and a follow-up study in 2000, researchers found that utilizing pictographs increased subjects' recall of verbal information from 17 to 85 percent (Houts et al., 1998; Houts, Witmer, Egeth, Loscalzo, & Zabora, 2000).

Teaching products may assist in instructing patients, but the need for a patient educator to help the patient receive and process information is vital. Multimedia, including video education, has potential to complement a patient educator's teaching efforts, especially with patients who are visual learners (Davis et al., 1998; Doak, Doak, & Root, 1995; Yancey, Tanjasini, Klein, & Tunder, 1995). For example, a randomized heart-failure study of 76 patients revealed that video education can assist in patient learning of symptom management but concluded that video education should be used as an adjunct to in-person education (Albert, Buchsbaum, & Li, 2007). Hill and colleagues found that in the population over 60 years of age, video instruction was slightly more effective for prevention of falls than an instruction book (Hill et al., 2009). Though multiple patient educational tools are available to complement a patient educator's instructional efforts, one major limitation of these tools is their inability to accommodate the unique needs and informational receptivity of the person receiving the information. Patients need a healthcare provider to help them as they try to grasp new information and merge it with their personal frame of reference for real-world application (Redman, 2004).

Cultural competence in healthcare is an issue that frequents the agendas of various professional and political groups (Dogra, Betancort, Park, & Sprague-Martinez, 2009) because cultural competencies address disparities in healthcare (Kleinman & Benson, 2006). The concept of cultural competence has been difficult to apply in the healthcare setting (Kleinman & Benson, 2006). Individual patient-centered education moves beyond cultural influence to personal being.

SUMMARY

- The approach to health literacy needs to move from being disease oriented to being patient oriented.

- There is a need to transition patient education from the global, standardized, one-size-fits-all model to an individually focused effort tailored specifically for each person.

- While healthcare providers may be a valuable source of information, more training may be needed to effectively educate patients.

- Today, even with all the technologic advances that have been achieved, especially in healthcare, the common task of communication of health information remains virtually undefined.

- Patient teaching can only be effective if the patient learns through meaningful dialogue and understands the information provided.

- People are living longer, they are living sicker, and they are living sicker longer. A shift toward increasing the autonomy of healthcare consumers could provide needed relief for our overburdened healthcare system.

- Teaching products may assist in instructing patients, but the need for a patient educator to help the patient receive and process information is vital.

- Patients need a healthcare provider to help them as they try to mentally grasp the new information and then merge it with their personal frame of reference for real-world application.

- Individual patient-centered education moves beyond cultural influence to personal being.

CHAPTER 3

Education Theory

There are two overarching theoretical education frameworks that serve to support the strategies used in the art and science of human learning: pedagogy and andragogy. These theoretical structures are thought to cover the process of educating humans across the life span. Francis Bacon believed in two types of learning: learning in children and learning in adults. Bacon spoke of pedagogy as the framing of morality. Adult learning, in Bacon's writings, is closely associated with religious beliefs and challenging mental faculties. Regarding adult learning, Bacon maintains we cannot teach people, we can only help them in their learning (Bacon, 1893). A review of pedagogy and andragogy theory can help a patient educator in approaching the initial stages of cultivating health knowledge with a patient.

PEDAGOGY

Pedagogy is derived from the Greek words *paid* (meaning *child*) and *agogus* (meaning *leader of*). In Latin, the term *pedagogue* means *teacher*. Pedagogy means the art and science of teaching children (Knowles, Holton, & Swanson, 2005). The pedagogic model of education is a set of principles that are based on assumptions of teaching and learning that evolved between the seventh and twelfth centuries in the monastic and cathedral schools of Europe through their experiences teaching young boys (Knowles, Holton, & Swanson, 2005). These traditional pedagogic curricula were grounded in social and political values, free of student ideology and discernment (Alexander, 2004). Didactic information, deemed socially relevant, was instilled into students through subject-oriented content. Pragmatism and conformity were cornerstones of the traditional curricula (Alexander, 2004).

In a pedagogic model, the learners' "need to know" is predetermined for them by the teacher (Knowles, 1984). The teacher is the axis of control for what students will be taught, how it will be taught, and what will constitute successful educational achievement (Hiemstra & Sisco, 1990). Learning is teacher planned, delivered, and directed in pedagogy. The student role is one of submissiveness and dependence on the teacher in the learning quest (Hiemstra & Sisco, 1990). External motivators such as grades, teacher approval, and parental pressure are familiar tools used in pedagogic learning.

   ## Case Study

Taylor, the local paperboy, is in the ninth grade at St. Joseph's Middle School. Recently, several town locals have spotted Taylor's mother, Joanie, delivering more papers on Taylor's paper route than Taylor. According to Ms. Haddie, Taylor and Joanie's next-door neighbor, Joanie is having Taylor spend more time on his algebra homework. Apparently Taylor is having great difficulty grasping the basics of algebra. St. Joesph's Middle School is a feeder school to St. Patrick's High School, which is a college preparatory school; Taylor has to make a "C" or better in ninth-grade algebra to qualify for admission to St. Patrick's. Taylor would prefer to take geometry because he did so well in it in eighth grade, but to meet St. Patrick's admission prerequisites he must successfully complete ninth grade algebra.

Expert Support for Action

Traditional pedagogic curricula are grounded in social and political values, free of student ideology and discernment (Alexander, 2004). Didactic information deemed relevant is instilled into students through subject-oriented content (Alexander, 2004). In a pedagogic model, the learners' "need to know" is predetermined for them by the teacher (Knowles, 1984). The teacher controls what will be taught, how it will be taught, and what will constitute successful educational achievement (Hiemstra & Sisco, 1990).

In the 19th century, when secular schools were established in the United States, the pedagogic model was used because it was the only known model of education (Knowles, Holton, & Swanson, 2005). Pedagogy assumptions served as the theoretical framework for all educational efforts, even for higher education that involved adults. For multiple generations, adults were taught using the same methodology as children. After World War I, assumptions about adult learning started to emerge (Knowles, Holton, & Swanson, 2005). These assumptions began to establish a foundation that would progress into an educational philosophy and would ultimately form the theoretical framework of andragogy.

ANDRAGOGY

The term *andragogy* comes from the Latin word *andr*, which means man. Andragogy is the art and science of helping adults learn (Knowles, Holton, & Swanson, 2005). Malcolm Knowles may be known as the father of andragogy, but he was not the first to coin the phrase. In 1833, the term *andragogy* was first introduced by a German schoolteacher, Alexander Kapp, who used the word to describe the educational theory of the Greek philosopher Plato (Knowles, Holton, & Swanson, 2005). A few years later, Johan Friedrich Herbart expressed his opposition to the word's use in the description of the great philosopher, which caused the term to fall out of favor and to disappear for nearly a hundred years. In 1921, the term resurfaced when it was used by Eugen Rosenstock, a social scientist who expressed his opinion that adult learners require a special teaching approach based on andragogy's unique methodology and philosophy (Knowles, et al., 2005). In 1951, Heinrich Hanselmann, a Swiss psychiatrist, published the book *Andragogy: Nature, Possibilities, and Boundaries of Adult Education,* which focused on the reeducation of adults. In 1956, 1957, and 1959, publications in academic and secular literary works thrust the term *andragogy* into mainstream use (Knowles, Holton, & Swanson, 2005).

In 1950, Malcolm Knowles published his first book, *Informal Adult Education,* which explicated the concept that adults learn best in informal, comfortable, flexible, nonthreatening settings. The groundbreaking work of Malcolm Knowles' theory of andragogy has helped add definition and focus to the art and science of adult learning. However, his work also sparked controversy in the world of academia.

Malcolm Knowles' assumptions were derived from studies done on the adult learner, primarily by Piaget and Erikson (Knowles, 1973, 1980). He proposes that as individuals mature into adults, their concept of self changes the manner in which they approach learning. Knowles' theory has six assumptions about the adult learner. Each of these assumptions easily translates into patient education in the healthcare setting.

According to Knowles (1975), adult learners:

- Need to know why they need to learn something
- Are self-directed and maintain responsibility for decisions and life events
- Bring a growing reservoir of experience that serves as a resource for learning in the educational activity
- Have a readiness to learn things they need to know to manage their life and real situations in their various social roles
- Are life-centered in their orientation to learning
- Are more responsive to internal motivators than external motivators

Knowles calls for educators to:

- Set a cooperative learning climate
- Create mechanisms for mutual planning
- Arrange for an analysis of learner needs and interests
- Establish learning objectives based on the identified learners' needs and interests
- Design sequential activities to achieve the objectives
- Execute the design by selecting varied methods, materials, and resources
- Evaluate the quality of the learning experience while diagnosing additional learning needs

In andragogic methodology, the instructor shifts from the pedagogic role of the source of information to that of a facilitator, an expert resource who helps guide the learner toward knowledge (Knowles et al., 2005). Educator and learner work together to meet mutually identified learning objectives. The learner helps establish the direction of instruction by communicating personally perceived knowledge-needs. Knowles used a five-point scale from low to high for learner self-evaluations (Knowles, 1975). In andragogy, the learner is self-directed, actively seeking and moving toward knowledge. The employment of various resources and methodologies assist the instructor in guiding the learner toward desired information (Knowles, 1950, 1975). Andragogy theory advocates for the educator-learner activity to be inclusive of learner value, life experience, and learner-identified needs in establishing the foundational structure for adult education.

Case Study

Jim, a local plumber, is a 48-year-old Caucasian male who has been diagnosed with diabetes mellitus. Jim has been attending local diabetes education classes and reading information published by the American Diabetes Association. Jim has progressed through grieving for the loss of his health and has accepted his diagnosis. Jim feels he needs to take control of his disease and is ready to resume power over his life. He has sought out information online and is actively participating in his diabetes class. Jim states that he is feeling stronger because he now understands how to carry out his daily care and why these actions are needed. Since Jim has assumed responsibility over his care, his blood glucose levels have remained stable within the targeted range established by his primary-care physician.

Understanding pedagogy and andragogy methodology can help establish capacity and context in education activities. Both philosophies bring forth various charges of teacher and learner, while offering external and internal influences affecting knowledge-gain in conventional education. Although both pedagogy and andragogy principles can be applied to any learning scenario, the unique influences encountered in the healthcare setting present a need to specifically focus on health education.

MEDAGOGY

Patients who misunderstand what their healthcare providers are trying to communicate to them can suffer devastating, and potentially fatal, consequences (Osborne, 2005). The treasure chest of assumptions from pedagogy and andragogy offer a good footing on the path to teaching patients and accommodating their learning needs. Challenges encountered by patient education activities cannot be met solely through customary academic approaches. It is necessary for patient educators to understand that each patient is a unique learner. The challenge is determining how healthcare providers can best structure information so each patient can receive it, understand it, remember it, and use it.

Medagogy offers a theoretical foundation that healthcare providers can use to construct a defined, methodical approach to patient education. Medagogy examines the process of patients' knowledge construction, acquisition, and proliferation as they move through the healthcare system (Stewart, 2009). Each healthcare provider serves as a source of health knowledge, while each patient serves as a source of self-knowledge. Both provider and learner have an active role in contributing to the progression of each other's knowledge.

It is a daily challenge for healthcare providers to educate people whose health statuses are virtually consuming their every thought. The charge of helping someone make a mental connection with critical information in a time of crisis is rare in traditional education but a normal occurrence in healthcare (Friberg, Andersson, & Bengtsson, 2007; McCabe, 2004). Information from the healthcare provider bears on the health, life, and welfare of the consumer of healthcare services: the patient. Information from the patient influences cost of care, inclusion of personal values, self-perceived ability, and health outcomes (Friberg, Andersson, & Bengtsson, 2007). Whether it is for preventive intercession or a reaction to insult or lifestyle, teaching a patient involves circumstances that are not regularly encountered in traditional education (Falvo, 2004; Friberg, Andersson, & Bengtsson, 2007; Redman, 2004).

When laypersons (patients) access the healthcare system, they are entitled to receive information regarding their health status and options for healthcare. Patients may present with health ranging from excellent to critical. In order to maximize resources to assist patients in attaining their health goals, providers must communicate via information exchange with patients; this is patient education. Medagogy focuses on the art and science of patient education by providing a conceptual framework for understanding the patient in the learning process (Stewart, 2009). The conceptual framework for medagogy is discussed in detail in Section 4.

SIGNIFICANCE TO HEALTHCARE

Patient teaching is a component of professional practice for healthcare providers (Boyd, Gleit, Graham, & Whitman, 1998). Patient education has been referred to as the "essence of nursing" (London, 1999, p. 7).

Healthcare providers serve as the perfect medium to help patients gain health independence, provide appropriate self-management, enhance treatment adherence, and improve overall health status (Friberg, Andersson, & Bengtsson, 2007; Henderson, 2002). Though healthcare providers are strategically positioned to assume the role of patient educator, not all providers have been adequately taught how to educate patients and their families. Luker and Caress (1988) targeted a large population of healthcare providers when they boldly asserted, "nurses are not good teachers" (p. 714). The inadequate performance of any healthcare professional as an educator may result from a lack of training in the skills of teaching or educating (Chang & Kelly, 2007; Luker & Caress, 1988). The lack of provider-training in the art of teaching only amplifies the problem of addressing patient knowledge, since the student in the healthcare setting is a patient.

The healthcare student (i.e., the patient) deals with multiple barriers to learning. Examples of possible barriers to patient learning include pain, fear of the unknown, separation from support systems such as family and friends, unfamiliar surroundings, and problems at home (for example childcare concerns). The sickness of the patient-student, not to mention the potentially fatal errors in self-care that can occur if patient learning is not achieved, makes patient education a challenge (Gabbay, Cowie, Kerr, & Purdy, 2000). Healthcare environments establish a teaching climate that does not parallel traditional academic settings. Figure 3-1 is a visual representation of two sick students and one healthy student.

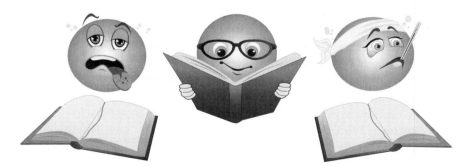

Figure 3-1. Three patient-students are reading. Two of the students are sick and distracted, while the healthy student is involved in reading the book he is holding. The figure serves to display the learning barrier that physical illness can present.

In healthcare, the patient educator has to make sure the patient can receive the information delivered. The patient's health status can interfere with reception of information, potentially acting as a barrier to learning and ultimately forestalling health promotion (Gabbay, Cowie, Kerr, & Purdy, 2000).

The World Health Organization and the European Commission Reports highlight that effective communication is critical to understanding health information (Stableford & Mettger, 2007). The Institute of Medicine (IOM), the Agency for Healthcare Research, and Health Association Libraries Section, a component of the Medical Library Association, have all produced reports that stress the need for clear, congruent, legitimate information for patients (Stableford & Mettger, 2007).

The practice of teaching healthcare providers to communicate information and evaluate patient understanding has not been a research priority for all healthcare professionals, but is needed to address the major concern of health literacy (Major & Homes, 2007). Where can patients get the information they need delivered according to learning principles and educational theories? Greenburg (2001), a health literacy expert, calls for health educators to whom healthcare providers can refer patients for education. The patient educator would help the patient understand his health status and treatment. Greenburg suggests that patient educators be used to teach healthcare information based on the individual patient's needs. Healthcare providers are in a unique position to provide the needed interpretation and information-accommodations for patients (Erlen, 2004). Greenburg refers to patient education as a new and evolving specialty that could become embedded into holistic patient care (Greenburg, 2001). Through good patient education, patients acquire the knowledge they need to cope with their disease, which can reduce mortality and morbidity and enhance a patient's quality of life (Cooper, Booth, Fear, & Gill, 2001). A patient's personal adaptation or psychological adjustment and acceptance should be of paramount concern to healthcare providers (Cooper et al., 2001).

The teaching styles of some healthcare providers create learning barriers (Tattersall, 1995), while other barriers such as fear and pain are common in healthcare (Smith, 2011; Bastable, 2006). Patient-provider communication can improve through evaluations of patient comprehension and by instructing providers on how to teach patients (Paasche-Orlow, Schillinger, Greene, & Wagner, 2006). People have varying learning styles and different literacy levels. Patient education needs to be designed to accommodate each individual's educational and cultural diversities and individual abilities (Curry, Walker, Hogstel, & Burns, 2005; Kurashige, 2008). Learning is an intricate, difficult, and demanding skill that needs to occur in a conducive environment (Bastable, 2006; Parikh, Parker, Nurss, Baker, & Williams, 1996).

In 1999, five categories for influencing the development and improvement of patient education were identified:

- healthcare organization,
- professional value,
- healthcare policy,
- evidence-based practice, and
- training and methodologic support (Deccache & Aujoulat, 2001).

Training and methodologic support refers to the education of healthcare providers in the multidimensional process of human learning (i.e., training providers to be educators). In an attempt to address the health knowledge needs of healthcare consumers, the Organization of Patient Educators (OPE) released a course that trains healthcare providers in andragogy and pedagogy, laws of learning, behavioral theories, and the theory of medagogy. The OPE certifies healthcare providers who complete the patient educator course, implement a patient teaching plan, and pass an intensive exam as Certified Patient Educators (CPEs). The information taught in the course is used every day in the practices of CPEs.

In the Centers for Medicare and Medicaid 9th scope of work's pilot-care transitions, the Louisiana Quality Initiative Organization (QIO) utilized the medagogy framework after OPE's training and credentialing of their CMS pilot employees. The medagogy model was the Louisiana QIO's unique approach to meeting established care-transitions pilot benchmarks. In 2010, the Louisiana QIO's Care Transitions work was acknowledged by CMS as the nation's most innovative healthcare project (Griggs, 2011; Johannessen, 2010).

SUMMARY

- There are two overarching theoretical education frameworks that serve to support the strategies used in the art and science of human learning—pedagogy and andragogy.
- Pedagogy means the art and science of teaching children.

- In pedagogy, learning is teacher planned, delivered, and directed. The student role is one of submissiveness and dependence on the teacher in the learning quest.
- Andragogy is the art and science of helping adults learn.
- In 1950, Malcolm Knowles published his first book, *Informal Adult Education*, which explicated the concept that adults learn best in informal, comfortable, flexible, and nonthreatening settings.
- The treasure chest of assumptions from pedagogy and andragogy offer a good footing on the path to teaching patients and accommodating their learning needs.
- It is necessary for patient educators to understand each patient as a unique learner.
- Medagogy offers a theoretical foundation that healthcare providers can use to construct a defined, methodical approach to patient education.
- Medagogy examines the process of patients' knowledge construction, acquisition, and proliferation as they move through the healthcare system. Both provider and learner have an active role in contributing to the progression of each other's knowledge in medagogy.
- The charge of helping someone make a mental connection with critical information in a time of crisis is rare in education, but is a normal occurrence in healthcare.
- The healthcare student (i.e., the patient) deals with multiple barriers to learning. Examples of possible barriers to patient learning include pain, fear of the unknown, separation from support systems such as family and friends, unfamiliar surroundings, and problems at home with childcare.
- In healthcare, the patient educator has to make sure the patient can receive the information delivered.
- The practice of teaching healthcare providers to communicate information and evaluate patient understanding has not been a research priority for all healthcare professionals, but is needed to address the major concern of health literacy.
- The teaching styles of some healthcare providers create learning barriers, while other barriers like fear and pain are common in healthcare.
- In an attempt to address the health knowledge needs of healthcare consumers, the OPE released a course that trains healthcare providers in

andragogy and pedagogy, laws of learning, behavioral theories, and the theory of medagogy. OPE certifies healthcare providers who complete the patient educator course, implement a patient teaching plan, and pass an intensive exam as CPEs.

- Medagogy offers the prospect of bringing the skill of patient education into an organized, interdisciplinary healthcare model used to educate each patient so their health literacy needs and healthcare goals can be adequately addressed.

SECTION I SUMMARY

In healthcare, the patient-provider relationship offers unique educational opportunities that are unlike the conditions that exist in any other institution. Each patient is a unique student with one-of-a-kind qualities and needs. Often, patients do not receive the information they need from healthcare providers. An accurate understanding of health-related information is needed for patients to partner with providers and for providers to partner with patients to achieve optimal healthcare goals and favorable outcomes. Healthcare providers need to diligently plan and carefully articulate the information patients need in order to be involved and active in their healthcare (Redman, 2003). Patients need to assert their healthcare goals and knowledge, which will help patients assume their rightful position in the planning and management of their treatment. Good patient education serves as a foundation for quality care (Tattersall, 1995). Patient education may cost more in advance, but ultimately the cost of care will be less and money will be saved (Tattersall, 1995). Patient education is a basic duty of healthcare providers. Successful patient education is a gift of knowledge that empowers individuals and families. Patients have the right to know so that they can make informed decisions and be in control of their healthcare (U.S. Department of Health and Human Services, 1999). Medagogy offers the prospect of bringing the skill of patient education into an organized, interdisciplinary healthcare model to be used to educate each patient so their health literacy needs and healthcare goals can be adequately addressed.

SECTION II

EFFECTIVE TEACHING AND LEARNING

[CHAPTER 4]

Information Exchange

Information is a powerful tool in the healthcare provider–patient relationship. This section focuses on definitions for teaching and learning as they relate to patient knowledge attainment. Teaching methodologies and theories assert beliefs about what happens in the teaching and learning process, although these methodologies and theories are usually associated with traditional educational settings (i.e., schools and colleges). This section is intended to expose the reader to information that can aid the healthcare provider and patient educator in mastering the teaching and learning process in the healthcare setting.

PATIENT-PROVIDER EXCHANGE OF INFORMATION

Personally possessing information can be a source of enlightenment regarding choices and potential opportunities, whereas lack of knowledge can cloud the decision-making process. People function within the limits of their knowledge. A lack of information can be detrimental to the quality of choices that are made (Hirsch, 1988). To completely capture the process of information delivery between health provider and patient, the information exchange must be explored from provider to patient and patient to provider. A narrow focus has long governed patient education and the patient's assumed gain of understanding from the provider (Mordiffi, Tan, & Wong, 2003). Patient education has focused on the provider's role in sharing knowledge with the goal of moving the patient forward in their health (Boyde et al., 2009; Hahn, 2009). Although providers educating patients may intend to increase patient understanding, they need to recognize their position as pupils of their patients in the provider-patient information exchange process (Safran et al., 1998; Weiner, Barnet, Chang, & Daaleman, 2005). This includes learning about the intricacies of their patients' personal lives. Providers need to gain understanding from information they receive from their patients (Hahn, 2009; Weiner, Barnet, Chang, & Daaleman, 2005).

Educator and learner roles constantly shift throughout provider-patient communication interactions. Just as healthcare decisions are made from information the patient receives from the provider, the provider also learns valuable information from the patient (Hahn, 2009). Providers use the details of the information the patient shares to assist in the construction and formulation of a treatment plan. The more insight the provider has, the more patient-specific the provider can be when rendering treatment options and participating in treatment planning (Boyde et al., 2009; Wakefield & Jorm, 2009; Weiner, Barnet, Chang, & Daaleman, 2005). The flow of information between the patient and healthcare provider is a fluid dynamic that perpetually stimulates change and action through choice for both receivers (Hahn, 2009).

In healthcare, there is a need for the patient-learner to receive instruction as well as to educate the provider about his personal experiences, values, and goals (Epstein et al., 2005; Hahn, 2009; Leonard & Wilijer, 2007). Likewise, a need exists for the healthcare provider to instruct the patient regarding knowledge of human health, healthy behaviors, and health options, as they simultaneously receive instruction from the patient. The more personal knowledge the provider gains about a patient, the better is the communication between the provider and the patient (Mordiffi, Tan, & Wong, 2003). Shared information between provider and patient will result in a progressive experience that will allow each to directly exert influence in treatment planning (Epstein et al., 2005; Leonard & Wilijer, 2007; Tang & Lansky, 2005). Allowing personal influence increases the likelihood of including individual preferences and values while moving toward optimal health (Kaufman, 2008; Shaw, Huebner, Armin, Orzech, & Vivian, 2009).

Knowledge is a source of power. Traditionally, the provider has assumed power in the provider-patient relationship (Epstein et al., 2005;

Leonard & Wilijer, 2007; Walford & Alberti, 1985). Influence in treatment has been limited to the healthcare provider's assertions and assumptions (Leonard & Wilijer, 2007; Mordiffi, Tan, & Wong, 2003). While the healthcare provider brings expert knowledge of health to the provider-patient relationship, too often what the patient brings to the relationship is overlooked, ignored, or assumed (Boyde et al., 2009; Mordiffi, Tan, & Wong, 2003). The patient provides his expert knowledge of self including personal values, experiences related to disease expression, personal needs, cultural beliefs related to health and illnesses, and desired outcomes (Leonard & Wilijer, 2007; Mordiffi, Tan, & Wong, 2003; Shaw, Huebner, Armin, Orzech, & Vivian, 2009). Without the information of self that the patient brings to the relationship, the patient is at risk for misdiagnosis, misappropriation of resources, and mismanagement of health (Collins, Gullette, & Schnepf, 2004; Swanson, 2007). The skills and knowledge from both the provider and patient, or the self-and the health-expert, is needed for the formation of an effective treatment plan that can achieve optimal health outcomes (Epstein et al., 2005).

SPAN OF INFLUENCE

Literature supports the relationship between knowledge and power (Bishop, 2009; Hutchinson, Hutchinson, & Arnaert, 2009; Rumsey, Hurford, & Cole, 2003; Simonton, 1985). This means that patients with more information have a greater ability to influence their healthcare. Span of influence is related to the understanding of information directly and indirectly associated with a given situation. Figures 4-1 and 4-2 visually display the relationship between knowledge gain and span of influence.

As the span of influence increases, the amount of direct effect a person can have over a situation enlarges. The wider the span of influence is, the greater the personal influence a person can exert in the planning and delivery of healthcare treatment. A large span of influence may be present but not used if a patient does not claim and exercise the power associated with the span of influence (Bishop, 2009; Longtin et al., 2010; Rumsey, Hurford, & Cole, 2003). The personal power connected with the span of influence must be asserted to influence the patient's treatment plan.

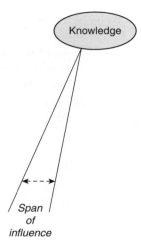

Figure 4-1. The span of influence is the area between the angled lines. The degree of area represented in the span of influence corresponds to patient knowledge.

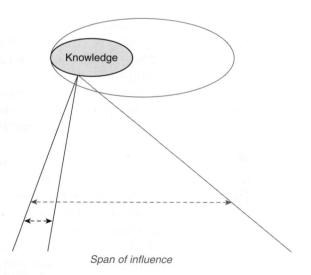

Figure 4-2. There is a positive relationship between expansion of knowledge and increased span of influence.

Case Study

Roger is a 52-year-old Asian male who entertains the community at public events as a musician. Roger admittedly tries to avoid healthcare providers as much as possible. As a child Roger had to visit his pediatrician and physical therapist often because of leg braces he had to wear to correct his genu varum (bow legs). He recalls his obstinacy to the leg-brace therapy and the lack of control he had in whether to use the prescribed treatment. This early interaction with the healthcare field left Roger with an overwhelming feeling of powerlessness as a patient. His impression of healthcare providers gained in early childhood has influenced his interaction with healthcare providers throughout his life. When Roger accesses healthcare he answers questions quickly and concisely. Roger tries to get a solution to what he perceives as a health issue in the quickest and least personal way. The healthcare provider offers a solution, and after the visit Roger decides if he will adhere to the provider's suggestion. Because Roger grew up feeling his opinion was not valued by the provider he has made healthcare an impersonal business transaction. Laughingly, Roger stated he has a better relationship with the self-serve gas station he uses than he does with his primary care provider. Roger firmly believes that his primary care provider does not even know he is a person, let alone his patient. The lack of relationship and effective communication between provider and patient led Roger to miss his follow-up visits after his last hospital stay for pneumonia. This interruption in the treatment course caused Roger's condition to exacerbate, and he was readmitted to the hospital only 20 days after his discharge. Roger lost time at work and his insurance had to pay for what should have been an avoidable hospital readmission.

Expert Support for Action

Fear and pain are common in the healthcare learning environment (Perry, 2006). Patients may also experience illness, emotions (e.g., anger, insecurity, and sorrow), financial insult, chaos, urgency, and more. It is easy to understand how learning can become very challenging in this environment (Levinson, Gorawara-Bhat, & Lamb, 2000; Rolls, Horrak, Wade, & McGrath, 1994). Fear, lack of control, and grieving for loss of health are all emotions that patients are likely to experience in healthcare (Jervey, 2001;

Mitchell, Murray, & Hynson, 2008). As discussed earlier, the provider has traditionally assumed power in the provider-patient relationship (Epstein et al., 2005; Leonard & Wilijer, 2007; Walford & Alberti, 1985). Influence in treatment has been limited to the healthcare provider's assertions and assumptions (Leonard & Wilijer, 2007; Mordiffi, Tan, & Wong, 2003). While the healthcare provider brings expert knowledge to the provider-patient relationship, too often the valuable information contributed by the patient is overlooked, ignored, or assumed (Boyde et al., 2009; Mordiffi, Tan, & Wong, 2003).

According to CMS, avoidable readmissions demands more than 12 billion in healthcare dollars annually (DeBrantes et al., 2010; Johannessen, 2010; Take steps, 2009,). Lack of patient understanding of their healthcare providers costs an annual price tag ranging between $160 and $236 billion annually (DeBrantes et al., 2010; Villaire & Mayer, 2009).

TEACHING

Teaching and learning is a dynamic and complex process that continues to impress and puzzle expert educators. From behaviorists to the evolving field of neurocognitive science, the teaching and learning process has yet to be completely understood (Wlodkowski, 2008). Though science may not ever completely grasp all that occurs in the teaching and learning process, there are many elements generally accepted as integral parts. Teaching, one of the oldest professions in the world, focuses on knowledge exchange. Plato's scholarly interactions with his students helped to establish teaching methodology that framed knowledge for generations beyond the protégés at his feet. Religious orders, such as monastics, committed their lives to improving society through education (Feldman & McPhee, 2008). Political equality movements used education to limit social distortion and remove barriers (Mondale & Patton, 2001; Nasaw, 1997). Through all the changes that have occurred in education, one constant has remained: knowledge is power. Knowledge offers control and enlightenment to the beholder. As Francis Bacon affirmed, knowledge serves as an intellectual map that helps one to choose the right path (Price, 1893). The art and science of teaching focuses on the act of delivering information designed to enlighten the receiver through knowledge acquisition and increased personal wisdom (Alexander, 2004; Knowles, Holton, & Swanson, 2005). Pring (2004) asserts that to teach is to engage intentionally in those activities that bring about learning.

Academia has evolved into the presently accepted setting for teaching and learning. Although teaching takes place in various settings, school in today's society is the traditional setting where teaching, instruction, and training are routinely performed. Public schools with mandated attendance have helped to condition members of society to automatically assume the role of student upon entry into an academic setting (Mondale & Patton, 2001; Nasaw, 1979). School settings are universally accepted as a resource for information and a destination for improved knowledge.

INTERNET

Today education is limitless, as it has progressed from the bricks and mortar of a schoolhouse to the unlimited access available from Internet connectivity. According to a 2001 Pew Internet and American Life Project, students are no longer pouring over pages for information after hours of searching a library; the convenience of the Internet has placed knowledge just a click away. The Internet provides a venue to conveniently access research for papers or schoolwork (Lenhart, Simon, & Graziano, 2001). Instant messaging and e-mail communication with peers and instructors can provide students with homework assistance in minutes (Lenhart, Simon, & Graziano, 2001). Web sites can serve as sources of information for students or projects for learning through web site construction (Lenhart, Simon, & Graziano, 2001). Computer technology with Internet access removes many traditional limitations and boundaries of education, offering powerful educational resources for the learners who are proficient in their utilization (Chang et al., 2004). Unfortunately, the population most affected by health decline and chronic illness, those age 65 and older, are caught in the "digital divide" either because of limited access or lack of Internet and computer usage knowledge (Campbell, 2008; Chang et al., 2004; Kaye, 2009). Commonly experienced effects of aging like decline in vision, hearing, and dexterity only add to the geriatric population's challenge in accessing advanced technology (Czaja & Lee, 2007). A 2009 report revealed that the geratric population is beginning to access the Internet more than they have in the past (Jones & Fox, 2009). Though this news is promising there is still much work that needs to be done in providing geriatric health Internet resources (Jones & Fox, 2009).

CENTEREDNESS OF INFORMATION AND INSTRUCTION

In healthcare, the heart and soul of any and every task and obligation is the patient. The same centeredness should carry over into patient education. One major duty of an educator is the identification of information that is prudent and beneficial for the learner to know. In the classroom, the teacher serves as the courier of information that faculty, administration, and academic standards have deemed prudent and beneficial for the learner to know. However, in healthcare the task of identifying prudent and beneficial information for the learner is not as planned and constructed. Healthcare has traditionally focused on the physical ailments and disorders of the body. However, to meet the patient's health needs, healthcare providers must concentrate on addressing the patient's knowledge and learning needs along with physical issues (Myers & Pelino, 2009).

Traditionally, the patient education encounter is educator-centered. The information that is taught is prioritized through the provider's knowledge of the patient's health status and a myriad of assumptions regarding the patient's life and values (Boyde et al., 2009). These assumptions could be clarified and validated with the patient but usually are not. This type of educator-centered instruction occurs when educators deliver information that they think the learner needs (Mordiffi, Tan, & Wong, 2003). Educator-centered instruction constructs information according to provider-oriented needs rather than patient-oriented needs and it reinforces the traditional segmenting of patients into disease or health states; information delivery should instead be formatted for the total patient. Patients should be taught holistically with information that reflects who they are and where they are in their personal health (Boyde et al., 2009). Information should be tailored toward each individual's "thumbprint" or one-of-a-kind knowledge needs (Boyde et al., 2009; Oliver, Kravitz, Kaplan, & Meyers, 2001).

Prefabricated patient-education products and third-party manufactured presentations contain disease-oriented information and serve as examples of educator-centered instruction because the individual patient is not included in the formation of these products. Instead, producers of these products work from assumptions about the potential receiver of the information. Individuality and personalization are removed from most conventional disease-oriented patient education materials. This is not to say that these products should not be used in healthcare; they can be used in a learner-centered teaching plan if they are complemented with a patient educator who frames the information to the patient's life

(Boyde et al., 2009; Mordiffi, Tan, & Wong, 2003). To be truly learner-centered, all instruction and teaching materials should be personalized to meet each individual patient's learning and knowledge needs (Bull, Kreuter, & Scharff, 1999; Falvo, 2004; Kyngas, 2003).

In order to address a patient's knowledge and learning needs in healthcare, an educator should construct a learner-centered plan for teaching. Learner-centered instruction focuses on issues and matters that are important to the learner. Ideally, the learner would help establish the prioritization of material to be taught by communicating their desired knowledge. Values, health goals, finances, and many other factors help influence the manner in which the patient receives, understands, and prioritizes information. Understanding the multitude of socioeconomic influences that patients experience can help a provider respect the choices patients ultimately make from the information the provider offers (Hahn, 2009).

Healthcare offers a unique situation in that needed knowledge may not be apparent to the learner. This lack of knowing is related to the healthcare provider's knowledge of health and treatment—the provider's healthcare expertise. The provider's expert knowledge is imperative in planning and prioritizing patient education. Learner-centered teaching in healthcare focuses all plans for education on the learner's needs, resources, individual knowledge, and health status (Hahn, 2009; Redman, 2006). If the learner does not recognize his learning deficits because of his lack of healthcare expertise, then the expert with that knowledge—the provider—must expose the learner to the information he lacks. The expert should be sensitive to the knowledge-deficits that the patient might be experiencing. Learner-centered teaching is planned through the partnering of provider and patient (Bensing, 2000; Boyde et al., 2009). This partnership offers an opportunity to construct a personalized teaching plan that is unique to each patient.

SITUATIONAL CENTEREDNESS

As previously noted, healthcare is not a traditional learning setting. Healthcare by its very nature creates this singular educational environment. Though learner-centered instruction is desirable, it is important to acknowledge that it is not always appropriate in the healthcare setting. Healthcare's unique milieu frequently requires situational-centered instruction because the challenges of illness, injury, and emergencies often leave the learner's situation in a volatile flux (Epstein et al., 2005). There are instances where healthcare decisions must be made within moments; in these instances, information has to be relayed as quickly as possible.

As a patient's health status stabilizes, information can shift into a learner-centered focus (Bensing, 2000). Healthcare environments require perpetual assessment on the part of the healthcare educator to know when the patient needs situation-centered information or learner-centered information. Centeredness of the information must be appropriate for the presenting health state (Bensing, 2000).

This present change in situation demands a strong commitment on the part of the provider to ensure that patient rights are always maintained as a priority (Falvo, 2004; Rankin & Stallings, 2001; Redman 2007). As discussed previously, patients have the right to make healthcare decisions. Patients' rights to information allow the patients to exert control over healthcare decisions while honoring their right to receive what they want from the healthcare provided (Rankin, Stallings, & London, 2005).

 Case Study

Transitioning the centeredness of patient education can be seen in the example of Steve, a 33-year-old Caucasian who is a chef at a fancy restaurant in town. Steve had a recent stay in the local acute-care hospital after he was injured by a rock thrown by a neighbor's lawn mower. The rock hit and became lodged in Steve's left eye. Steve was rushed to the local emergency department. Immediately Steve and his family were offered information regarding Steve's status and his need for surgery. Due to the sensitivity of the situation and the need to act swiftly, information was clear, concise, and direct. The information was centered according to the situation, which required immediate attention. Steve went through his surgery and remained an inpatient for two days.

During Steve's stay at the hospital, his patient education from the unit staff focused on things he needed to know as he transitioned to home, including:

- Medications

- Follow-up appointments

- Infection control methods

- Dressing change procedure

- Signs and symptoms of infection

The information was also inclusive of what Steve felt was important, including:

- Who to call if he has an issue
- What to do if he forgets to take his medication
- When he can go back to his normal routine and, most of all, when he can return to work

Every member of the staff added some piece of knowledge to Steve's health understanding, and before assuming Steve felt ready to care for himself the hospitalist, Dr. Badu, asked Steve how he felt about his ability to carry out his care independently. Dr. Badu's focus on the patient's comfort with assuming self-care duties as well as the staff's dedication to making sure Steve received the information he needed along with the information he wanted offered a more patient-centered approach to his patient education than had been done presurgery in the emergency department.

Expert Support for Action

The patient provides his expert knowledge of self, including but not limited to personal values, experiences related to disease expression, personal needs, cultural beliefs related to health and illnesses, and desired outcomes (Leonard & Wilijer, 2007; Mordiffi, Tan, & Wong, 2003; Shaw, Huebner, Armin, Orzech, & Vivian, 2009). Without the information about self that the patient brings to the relationship, misdiagnosis, misappropriation of resources, and mismanagement of health can occur (Collins, Gullette, & Schnepf, 2004; Swanson, 2007). The skills and knowledge from both the patient and provider, or the self and health expert, is needed for the formation of an effective treatment plan that will achieve optimal health outcomes (Epstein et al., 2005).

TRANSMITTING AND RECEIVING INFORMATION

While educators can deliver information, they do not possess power over knowledge acquisition; they cannot make someone learn (Ormrod, 2008). Likewise, the receiver or student does not completely control the reception and retention of information (Jensen, 2000) because the entire learning process is dependent on many variables. In order for the teaching effort to be effective, the information or content has to make a connection with the receiver. Educators attempt to match the delivery method so that the receiver's reception is improved and long-term storage of information is probable (Jensen, 2000; Ormrod, 2008).

SUMMARY

- Information is a powerful tool used in the healthcare provider–patient relationship.
- Though providers educating patients may intend to increase patient understanding, they need to recognize their position as pupils of their patients in the provider-patient information exchange process. This includes learning about the intricacies of their patients' personal lives.
- Educator and learner roles constantly shift throughout provider-patient communication interactions.
- The more personal knowledge the provider gains about a patient, the better is the communication between the provider and the patient.
- Knowledge is a source of power. Traditionally, the provider assumed power in the provider-patient relationship. Too often what the patient brings to this relationship is overlooked, ignored, or assumed.
- In healthcare, the heart and soul of any and every task and obligation is the patient. The same centeredness should carry over into patient education.
- Educator-centered instruction constructs information according to provider-oriented needs rather than patient-oriented needs.
- Prefabricated patient education products and third-party manufactured presentations contain disease-oriented information and serve as examples of educator-centered instruction because the individual patient is not included in the formation of these products.
- To be truly learner-centered, all instruction and teaching materials should be personalized to meet each patient's learning and knowledge needs.

- If the learner does not recognize his learning deficits because of a lack of healthcare expertise, then the expert with that knowledge (the provider) must expose the learner to the information the learner lacks.

- Although learner-centered instruction is desirable, it is important to acknowledge that in healthcare it is not always appropriate.

[CHAPTER 5]

The Science and Theories of Learning

Learning involves the act of receiving and storing information for future access. Hirsch (1988) defines knowledge as a network of information possessed by the learner that empowers the learner to obtain, process, and store new information. The learner must make a logical intellectual connection with the information the educator is offering for learning to transpire (Hess & Tate, 1991; Rice & Okun, 1994). For example, a student that does not know numbers cannot learn geometry; a baseline of knowledge must be present to build on. For the student to learn geometry he must know numbers and the order in which the numbers fall so he can appreciate the value of each number. A lack of foundational knowledge prohibits the opportunity for connecting known information with newly acquired information (Santrock, 2008; Zull, 2006). Without the foundational information, the new information may be remembered, but the learner will lack depth, fluidity, and ultimately solid understanding (Ormrod, 2008: Zull, 2006) because the student is missing the reasoning, or the "why," behind the new information.

A knowledge foundation provides a site on which to build additional information. Information must be ordered logically for the brain to be able to receive, process, and ultimately store it (Noddings, 2006). Logical ordering helps a learner sort, label, and catalog information for future retrieval (Pring, 2004; Rice & Okun, 1994), as well as simplify the assimilation and storage of new information (Kessels, 2003). An example of logical order is 1, 2, 3, 4, 5, or A, B, C; whereas, 4, 1, 3, 5, 2, or C, A, B would represent illogical or lack of order.

INSTRUCTIONAL METHODOLOGY FOR OPTIMAL LEARNING

Because information bears such significant influence in the provider-patient relationship, providers should see the delivery of information as a high priority. Preparing patient information so it can be well received helps ensure that patients have a better opportunity to participate and ultimately drive the direction of their healthcare. Planning and preparing patient information, just as a teacher plans and prepares information for students, offers an opportunity for healthcare providers to capitalize on proven academic techniques that can improve the possibility that the receiver—the patient—is successful in understanding the information delivered (Atherton, 2009; Ormrod, 2008; Sousa, 2006).

In academia, educators choose content that students need to know as well as the method of delivery for that content. The educator's goal in choosing the method of delivery should be to use methods that promote learning, best engage the learner, and facilitate the learner's mental connections that are necessary for understanding to occur (Sousa, 2006). Selecting a method of delivery in healthcare could include choosing between a lecture and a demonstration. It would benefit the provider to know that a lecture on how to do a fingerstick for glucose monitoring would not be as effective as watching a demonstration of someone performing the task (Sousa, 2006). According to Atherton (2009), lectures result in 5% mental retention after 24 hours. Demonstration, on the other hand, has a 30% retention rate after 24 hours. Immediately using learned information could boost the retention rate up to 90% (Ormrod, 2008; Sousa, 2006).

Packaging information for delivery can present a challenge for educators, especially in healthcare. Information should be delivered in a way that allows learners to best receive, process, and store the information (Ormrod, 2008). According to Pring (2004), regardless of the method of delivery chosen to communicate the information to the learner, all teaching activities should have the following in common:

- Intention to influence knowledge through learning
- Connection between what is presented and what is to be learned
- Connection between what is taught and the learner's presenting knowledge

The best method of delivery of information depends on what is right for the patient. In addition, educators must choose methods that correlate with their own personal skills and proficiencies. An educator who lacks competent teaching skills may interfere with the patient's assimilation and storage of information (Feldman & McPhee, 2008; Ormrod, 2008). Therefore, the method selected for information delivery should be both learner centered and educator mastered.

Currently, most patient education is done one-on-one at bedside or chairside or in classes with other patients. If a patient needs assistance with care or needs support, then family or significant others may also be included in patient learning sessions. One-on-one instruction offers an opportunity for the educator to construct and deliver information suited to the patient's individual needs. Too often in healthcare, the education patients receive ends up being either a formulaic presentation that is offered to every patient with a certain condition or an "oh-and-you-need-to-know" off-the-cuff delivery.

Many times the one-on-one teaching sessions are at the convenience of the educator and do not coincide with optimal timing for the patient. For example, consider a tired patient in a diabetic teaching session right after finishing a two-hour physical therapy session late in the afternoon in a rehabilitation hospital. The timing is perfect for the dietitian's schedule as she closes out her workday. However, it is less than optimal for the patient, who is tired. Preplanning and asking the patient what time would be best for their learning could help the provider and patient get their education sessions in sync (Redman, 2006).

Sometimes learning opportunities present themselves and then, shortly, the teachable moment has passed. These teachable moments are excellent in revealing where the patient is in their desire for knowledge (Falvo, 2004). These moments can initiate a fruitful learning experience because they offer the educator insight into the patient's knowledge priorities, allowing the educator to answer and address extraneous concerns that may have been overlooked because of relevance only to that particular patient. These serendipitous teaching moments also allow the educator to display a commitment to meeting the patient's personal knowledge needs by immediately providing attention to the patient's informational request (Redman, 2006). The information that is exchanged in these sessions should be included in the patient's teaching plan and become part of the patient's learning history (Falvo, 2004; Rankin, Stallings, & London, 2005).

Scheduled one-on-one teaching sessions can allow the patient to contribute to the direction of the teaching interaction. Educators must be open and encourage the patient to identify and share their self-diagnosed knowledge needs (Hahn, 2009; Tang & Lansky, 2005). Offering choice to the patient allows the patient control in his personal health education.

The more input the patient has in the selection of material to be covered, the more the patient stands to gain in knowledge and control (Coates, 2007). Allowing personal interests and preferences into the interaction provides an opportunity to cultivate deeper understanding and empowerment in patients (Stone, Pound, Pancholi, Farooqi, & Khunti, 2005; Tang & Lansky, 2005).

CONSCIOUS AND UNCONSCIOUS LEARNING

Jensen (2000) noted that only 10% of learning is conscious (explicit) while the remaining 90% is unconscious (implicit) (Shanks, 2010). The brain is such an amazing organ that it initiates learning before learning is consciously initiated (Jensen, 2000). Unconscious, or implicit, learning absorbs information from the whole picture through the use of sights, smells, and sounds (Jensen, 2000; Shanks, 2010). Jensen (2000) explains that implicit learning is learning through the body. The learner begins to internalize data on an unconscious level even before the first piece of planned information is formally delivered. Figure 5-1 displays the areas of

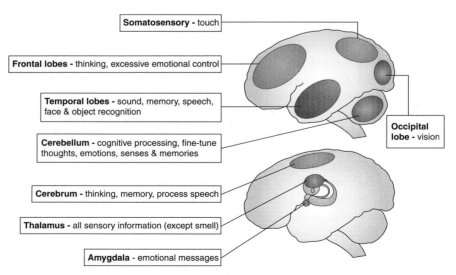

Figure 5-1. The various areas of the brain involved in information processing and storage for implicit learning (Sousa, 2006).

the brain that are used during implicit learning (Sousa, 2006). Understanding the brain's amazing abilities to learn can help educators as they plan educational sessions.

Knowing that the learning environment—from sounds to tactile sensations—play a part in the learner's ability to process information can help the educator prepare a plan that ensures the intended message is received and reinforced. Educators should strive to establish an optimal learning situation so they can maximize what is captured in the conscious (explicit) 10% of learning. A screaming, crying patient in the hall can negatively impact a message focused on teaching a preoperative patient effective pain control. Senses are stimulated as the learner hears sounds of screaming and crying, and emotions are triggered as the patient is concerned with approaching surgery and likely fearful of imminent postoperative pain. Unless a written form accompanies the verbal information, retention may be compromised because the senses are hyperstimulated, moving the focus of conscious attention to the sensual information coming in from the environment.

To ensure that the patient will learn the information intended to be communicated in a planned learning moment, the educator needs to capture the student's attention (Feldman & McPhee, 2008). Experience has taught that the patient educator needs to persuade or move the intended learner, the patient, into a state that is receptive to learning. Conscious learning is a voluntary state of attention focusing on prescribed information. The information may be new or associated with, similar to, or a reminder of information previously learned. In order to motivate the learner to move into a conscious learning state, the teacher or educator must gain the learner's interest by leading them to awareness. This can occur in several different ways (Feldman & McPhee, 2008). Movement into a learning consciousness happens after engagement occurs. Engagement includes mental and physical awareness and appeal. The mental and physical attraction facilitates concentration on the information being delivered. Engagement prioritizes information so that it mentally and physically limits personal attention toward other environmental options, while centering attention on information being conveyed. Once the receiver is engaged with the deliverer, then a concentrated effort on learning can occur.

To engage a learner, the provider might pose a provocative question to help the learner position a mental stance while ascertaining information related to the question. This stimulates interest in what is being said, and at the same time stimulates thinking (Feldman & McPhee, 2008).

Staggering statements like "40% to 80% of what a healthcare professional says is forgotten almost immediately" (Kessels, 2003) and profound or famous quotes such as "We will either find a way or make one" both offer the opportunity to capture the learner's attention (The Motivating Tape Company, 2000). A story of a problem, empirical data that supports possible outcomes, and personal experiences can also serve as attention-getters (Feldman & McPhee, 2008).

Engaging a learner also involves a concerted physical effort to show the learner that they are your present focus. The educator needs to get on the same physical level, facing the learner eye to eye and heart to heart (Boothman, 2002). A person who is in front of you and talking directly to you while looking you in the eye can grab your attention. Educators need to speak with compassion, concern, and confidence as they teach. The patient educator needs to humanize the information and personalize it so patients can easily fit it into their individual worlds. Casual conversation and active listening on the part of the educator can help in the extraction of information that can be used in the personalization of material to be taught. The more that is known about the person, the more the information can be personalized (Boothman, 2002).

Knowing the patient's level of knowledge on a topic is beneficial for constructing and planning what information needs to be delivered. Simple discussion with probing questions can help an educator gain insight into a patient's knowledge of their condition. For example, the healthcare provider might say, "Tell me about congestive heart failure, what is it?" Other methods can be used, like "test by discussion," which offers social interaction while providing relevant personal information. Patients will vary in their levels of receptivity; some will take longer to understand while others may not understand at all. The celebration of human learning honors the uniqueness of each individual in the learning process. Patience and skillful reframing of information for patient clarity can be very beneficial attributes of a patient educator. Once a patient's understanding of information is gained then the caregiver can determine how to communicate more information to them.

LEARNING DOMAINS

In the 1950s, Benjamin Bloom identified learning domains that include six levels of human thought which differ in complexity (Bloom, 1956). Each level of thought is dependent on the preceding level for successful accomplishment (Ormrod, 2008). Bloom's work illustrates the mental construction that human thought must complete to reach higher levels of understanding (Krathwohl, Bloom, & Masia, 1964). Autonomy and personal definition are achievable with stair-step maneuvering of knowledge up through the learning domains.

Bloom organized his cognitive levels into a taxonomy that many educators use in the construction of educational learning goals and objectives. Bloom's taxonomy assists educators in identifying where students need to be in their cognitive mastery of the information, while providing direction for increasing the complexity of knowledge. In 2001, Anderson and colleagues revised Bloom's taxonomy to incorporate theoretical advances that have been made in education. The revision transitioned the taxonomy into a two-dimensional framework, including six cognitive levels and four types of knowledge. Anderson and colleagues identified the four types of knowledge as factual, conceptual, procedural, and metacognitive (Anderson et al., 2001). Bloom's taxonomy can help educators better plan and strategically target their teaching efforts to assist students in their mastery of knowledge. Understanding the levels of knowledge can help the patient educator move the patient from the level of *remember* to *apply*.

  ### Case Study

Mr. Boudreaux is a 67-year-old Cajun fisherman who has peripheral vascular disease (PVD). Mr. Boudreaux has been told for years that he needs to elevate his feet. He can repeat past instruction without error. He fully complies with the limitations of no crossing legs, no elastic binding socks, and no tight underwear or pants. Mr. Boudreaux demonstrates that he remembers and understands the information. Recently, Mr. Boudreaux was assigned to a new post at his job. The new position requires Mr. Boudreaux to be in a harness that wraps around his waist and thighs and lifts him in the air. After two days in the new position Mr. Boudreaux was experiencing such leg pain and swelling that he had to see the company nurse, Donna. Even though Mr. Boudreaux has been the model patient in hearing and following his provider's advice, Mr. Boudreaux did not grasp the reason behind things he was told to do. Mr. Boudreaux could not apply the treatment rule of "avoid any constriction of circulation in your legs" to the harness he was wearing for his new position. Mr. Boudreaux was not able to see the harness as a means of constricting circulation in his legs. Helping Mr. Boudreaux master the ability to apply this rule independently should be the provider's focus for Mr. Boudreaux's education. Recognizing Mr. Boudreaux's inability to apply the treatment instruction to avoid circulatory constriction impelled Donna to explain to Mr. Boudreaux the PVD disease process. Donna then reviewed the symptoms that can occur, such as leg pain and swelling, while correlating the symptoms back to Mr. Boudreaux's presenting complaints. Mr. Boudreaux explained that he understood what happened. Frustrated, he went on to explain that he did not know how he would be able to always recognize things that could cause this to happen. Donna took an oblong balloon and blew it up half way, and then she pushed on one end forcing the air to move toward the other end. She then pushed on the opposite end forcing air back to the other side. She asked Mr. Boudreaux, "Do you see how easy the air moves in the direction I want it to?" Mr. Boudreaux says, "Of course." She hands the balloon to Mr. Boudreaux and has him manipulate the balloon by forcing air to shift side to side like she did. Then Donna applied pressure to the center of the balloon and asked Mr. Boudreaux to shift the air to the other side. Mr. Boudreaux applies pressure and states that he doesn't want to pop it as he makes the air shift to the other side. Donna then says, "Wasn't as easy to make the air move, was it? "No" states Mr. Boudreaux, "not while you are pinching it." Donna then compares the balloon to Mr. Boudreaux's leg. She goes on to explain that the pinching is a form of constriction. Just like the air shifted to one side and stayed on that side while she was pinching the balloon, the same thing happens when blood flow in the legs has something pinching or constricting the blood flow. The blood will stay on one side and swell because it is too hard for the body to push the blood through the pinched area. Mr. Boudreaux said, "Oh, so I need to think of my legs like a balloon." "Absolutely, you are correct" answered nurse Donna. "Always remember that anything tightly grabbing an area of your leg can cause the blood flow to be restricted, which will cause swelling. So yes, Mr. Boudreaux, think of your legs as balloons and avoid 'pinching.'"

Expert Support for Action

Without foundational knowledge, new information may be remembered, but there is no depth, fluidity, and ultimately no solid understanding (Ormrod, 2008: Zull, 2006). Aristotle (2009) asserts that within the understanding of "why" lies reason, which provides an insight or wisdom that can be used beyond the immediate intended utility. Understanding "why" helps establish a foundational rationale, which can be an asset in treatment decisions for both the provider and patient (Tokarz, 2009). When behavior modification is hoped for, providing a "why" up front can ease the discomfort and confusion associated with lack of access to, and therefore lack of understanding of, the full picture (Jensen, 2000; Redman, 2007).

LEARNING STYLES

Teaching and learning are intensely personal activities; not all teachers are the same and, more importantly, not all learners are the same. For teachers to be able to convey the desired information to the pupil, they must be able to meet each learner's distinct needs (Brookfield, 2006). Educators should attempt to personalize the design and delivery of information to accomplish this objective (Avillion, 2009).

Knowing a person's learning style enables the educator to tailor the delivery of information to the learner's preferred (and most effective) learning style. There are three types of perceptual processing learning styles: visual, tactile, and auditory (Avillion, 2009). According to Minninger (1997), approximately 55% of the general population are visual learners. Visual learners use the sense of sight to facilitate their mental ingestion of information. Seeing information helps aid visual learners in processing and retaining. Visual learners prefer to see illustrations, graphics, color, and even the instructor (Avillion, 2009).

The second most common learning style is tactile, which is also referred to as kinesthetic (Minninger, 1997). An estimated 30% of the population favors the kinesthetic learning style (Minninger, 1997). This type of learner is commonly referred to as a "doer." Learners that are "doers" are hands-on learners and are best able to process information through experiencing it via action or feeling. Physical movement as well as handling and manipulating items can assist these learners in knowledge absorption (Avillion, 2009).

Verbal or auditory learning is the third learning style. It is favored by 15% of the population (Minninger, 1997). These learners need to speak, read aloud, discuss, or explain information in an effort to process the knowledge through auditory stimuli (Avillion, 2009). Auditory learners best receive and remember information that is heard. These learners might appear to be uninterested in what is being communicated, when in fact they are actively listening (Avillion, 2009).

Material delivered according to a personal learning style can help the learner receive and process the information with ease, while increasing the likelihood for overall success in the learner's educational experience (Tuan, 2011; Anonymous, 2009; Feldman & McPhee, 2008; Costa et al., 2007). Unfortunately, knowledge of a person's learning style is not always available. Many healthcare admission forms ask patients their preference for receiving information, but people do not always know what learning style they favor or what learning styles could yield the best results for them. An answer to the question does not necessarily mean the delivery mode chosen by the patient accurately identifies their learning style.

A mixed approach of teaching can help an educator tap into all learning preferences in information delivery (Jensen, 2000). This approach incorporates all teaching and learning styles and can aid in delivery by exposing the student to information via each learning sense. Using teaching methods that accommodate multiple learning styles ensures that the learner's personal learning preference is included in delivery (Avillion, 2009). If mixed learning styles cannot be used because of the nature of the material being taught, the teaching setting, or the teaching method, then targeting the most common learning styles can offer a greater chance of success.

 Case Study

Jan, a physician assistant, plans to teach her patient Mike about his cholesterol. Upon admission, Mike, a 32-year-old welder, identified reading as his favorite way to receive information. In addition, Jan noticed that Mike had a crossword puzzle book in his hand. Because Mike listed "building projects" as a hobby and appears very inquisitive about his treatment, Jan has prepared a print-out of material she plans to review—one for her and one for Mike. She also has props including a piece of water hose, blue cotton balls, red cotton balls, and a crossword puzzle to use in their scheduled training session. Jan verbally reviews with Mike the information they will cover in their session today. Then Jan begins to read from the handout sheet while Mike follows along on his sheet. After reading the handout Jan begins to use her props, the hose and colored cotton balls, to visually show Mike the impact of plaque (red cotton balls) buildup in the arteries (hose). Jan even has Mike put the red cotton balls in the hose. Jan uses the blue and red cotton balls to show the desired relationship of good and bad cholesterol. After many laughs and questions, Mike states that he never knew his garden hose could help save his life and that now he really understands how important his cholesterol is to his health. Jan then gives Mike a crossword puzzle that uses all the information they reviewed today and tells Mike he has homework. Mike briefly glances at the puzzle and says that he will have it done before she comes back to see him again. Jan gathers her props and tells Mike that she will return in a couple of hours to check on him and retrieve his homework. Mike appeared to have enjoyed the instruction while Jan was able to communicate very important information to him. Jan's ability to use mixed teaching methods tapping into all learning styles is evident by the following:

- Auditory: discussion, verbal exchange, reading material out loud

- Kinesthetic: patient physically putting cotton ball in hose, laughing, crossword puzzle

- Visual: use of props, colored cotton balls, crossword puzzle, written material

Expert Support for Action

Studies show that individualized instructions increase comprehension and memory more effectively than standardized instructions (Morrow et al., 2005; Robinson, Callister, Berry, & Dearing, 2008). There are three types of perceptual processing learning styles: visual, tactile, and auditory (Avillion, 2009). Healthcare providers need to present information in a manner each patient can understand, recall, and use in their life and healthcare choices (Stableford and Mettger, 2007). A mixed approach of teaching can help an educator tap into all learning preferences in information delivery (Jensen, 2000). Using teaching methods that accommodate multiple learning styles ensures that the learner's personal learning preference is included in delivery (Avillion, 2009).

OVERLAP BETWEEN TEACHING AND LEARNING

Once information is received, the work of understanding and learning begins (Brookfield, 2006; Jones, 2000). Teachers can present information, but the assimilation of the material offered is the work of the student or receiver. Just as the teacher has been charged with the task of teaching, the receiver or student bears the responsibility of accepting, internalizing, and ultimately learning the information (Demetriou & Raftopoulos, 2005). Recognizing the inherently interdependent relationship of the concepts *teach* and *learn* along with the fact that both teacher and learner have to work to make knowledge delivery and assimilation occur, it is easy to conclude that the process of knowledge gained through instruction is a shared function between the teacher and the learner.

LEARNING THEORIES

In learning, knowledge and understanding are gained through study, instruction, or experience. Learning is a science. From neuron firing to schemata filing, many theories have tried to explain the process of learning, but just as no two fingerprints are the same, such is each individual experience in learning. At best, words can only serve to point out common threads in beliefs associated with the process of learning. In an attempt to provide a conceptual framework to the process of traditional education, multiple theories have evolved. Theories of learning attempt to explain how learning occurs (Knowles, Holton, & Swanson, 2005). The following section reviews learning theories.

There are three prominent theoretical views that hold sway in education regarding how learning occurs and the factors that influence learning: behaviorism, cognitivism, and constructionism. Although some educators are committed to one primary philosophy and choose to label themselves as a member and a practicing party of a particular theoretical belief, the process of learning is so uniquely personal that a broad knowledge of theoretical perspectives and their complements to the field of education can better serve an educator (Feldman & McPhee, 2008). When humans are involved, one recipe rarely, if ever, can serve all (Falvo, 2004; Redman, 2006). Therefore, patient educators should not conform to a single educational theory, but should instead understand the theories' underlying dogma and amalgamate parts that can complement the personal practice of the patient educator. The following theories are considered influences of medagogy.

Behaviorism

Behaviorists define learning as a change in behavior due to experience and the creation of habits, and see the mind metaphorically as an empty container (Feldman & McPhee, 2008). Behaviorists believe that human learning can only be explained through observable behaviors (Skinner, 1974; Thorndike, 1911). According to behaviorists, people act only as they are conditioned, and they believe that learning is only induced through external forces via conditioning (Baum, 2005; Skinner, 1991).

The theory of behaviorism asserts that all human behavior, from emotions to reasoning, can be explained and predicted through associations between external stimulations and the response to these stimuli (Feldman & McPhee, 2008; Hilgard, 1988; Pavlov, 1927; Skinner, 1974, 1991; Thorndike, 1911). Reflexive and automatic associations are known as classical conditioning (Pavlov, 1927; Watson, 1930). In the health care setting, it is normal for patients to become anxious when they are seeing a provider, a phenomenon commonly referred to as "the white coat syndrome" (Engler, 2005; Harlan, 2007; Kerr, 2008). The white coat syndrome is the result of negative stimulation or experiences recurring in a healthcare setting. For example, a child receiving a shot every time he visits a physician will eventually associate the physician with pain. In time, the mere mention of the physician may stimulate a sense of fear (see Figure 5-2).

Edward Thorndike authored three behaviorism laws that fall under the umbrella of his connectionism theory. According to connectionism, learning is the result of associations formed between stimuli and responses (S-R) (Ormrod, 2008; Thorndike, 1911, 1932; Thorndike; Bregman, Tilton, & Wood, 1928). Strong associations or "habits" can be strengthened or weakened depending on character—positive or negative—and regularity of exposure associated with S-R pairings (Lefrancois, 1995; Kearsley, 2009; Ormrod, 2008). As illustrated in Figure 5-2, the regular stimulus of a shot during physician visits yields a negative response of pain that eventually creates a mental association between visits and pain. Thorndike found that certain responses dominated others (Lefrancois, 1995; Kearsley, 2009; Thorndike, 1911, 1932; Thorndike et al., 1928). He noted that satisfying rewards directly influenced the frequency of behavior,

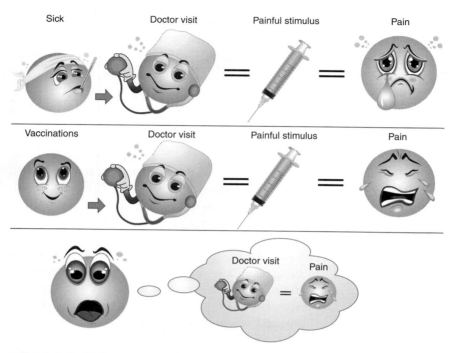

Figure 5-2. Mental associations can be formed from the consistent introduction of a painful stimulus such as an injection during a doctor's office visit. In health or illness, if a painful stimulus is consistently introduced, then a mental association between a physician's visit and pain can occur. Once the association is established, just the thought of a physician's visit can trigger thoughts of pain.

whereas discomforting or punishing rewards decreased behavior (Kearsley, 2009; Ormrod, 2008). The S-R theory evolved out of trial and error learning, which Thorndike identified as the most basic form of learning (Thorndike, 1911, 1932; Thorndike et al., 1928).

Thorndike asserted that neural connections were formed in response to perceived stimulus and the resulting response (Thorndike, 1911, 1932). He referred to the neural connections in the brain associated with the S-R pairing as "stamping in" (learning) and "stamping out" (forgetting) (Knowles et al., 2005; Ormrod, 2008; Thorndike, 1911; Thorndike et al., 1928). Thorndike recognized that humans and animals learn in a similar fashion, that learning is incremental, and that a person's readiness to learn is directly proportionate to the success of their learning experience (Bash,

2005; Hoare, 2006; Knowles et al., 2005). Three primary laws born from Thorndike's connectionism theory are the law of effect, the law of readiness, and the law of exercise (Bower & Hilgard, 1981; Kearsley, 1996; Merriam & Caffarella, 1991). The law of effect states that recurrence of responses is strengthened or weakened by its consequence or reward (Ormrod, 2008; Thorndike et al., 1928). The law of readiness maintains that if a sequence of responses known to yield a certain desired outcome is blocked, it will result in annoyance, which may diminish the student's level of desire to learn (Kearsley, 1996; Knowles et al., 2005; Thorndike et al., 1928). The law of exercise asserts that S-R connections that are repeated are strengthened, while S-R connections that are not used are weakened (Bower & Hilgard, 1981; Merriam, & Caffarella, 1991; Thorndike et al., 1928). Thorndike's three laws continue to exert major influence in human learning and the application of new behaviors.

Modifying behavior through learning is known as operant conditioning. The term operant (or instrumental) conditioning was coined by B.F. Skinner (Ormrod, 2008; Skinner, 1966, 1984). Skinner asserted that conditioning in behavior occurs because of rewards or punishments that happen in response to behavior (Ormrod, 2008; Watson, 1930). Behaviorists maintain the validity of three principles (Baum, 2005). Each of these laws complement each other. The first principle states that predictable links exist between a stimulus and the response it yields (Pavlov, 1927; Skinner, 1974, 1991; Thorndike, 1911; Watson, 1930). The second principle contends that through study and manipulation of conditions that influence behavior, behavior can be shaped and predicted with a high degree of certainty in a specific situation (Skinner, 1974, 1991). The final principle states that varied reinforcement can strengthen or weaken learned behavior (Feldman & McPhee, 2008; Pavlov, 1927; Thorndike, 1911; Watson & Rayner, 1920). Many weight-loss programs use behaviorism to modify member behavior. Members weigh in during support meetings. Weight loss is celebrated with rewards, while weight gain may involve negative consequences such as increased cost or possibly even dismissal from the program. The use of rewards and punishments helps condition or train the behavior of members to meet desired goals (Pavlov, 1927; Skinner, 1974, 1991; Thorndike, 1911; Watson, 1930).

Implications for the practice of patient education derived from the behaviorism theory center around behaviorists' belief that knowledge is not something that exists in the mind, but instead works as a form of guidance formed from actions (Baum, 2005; Feldman & McPhee, 2008; Watson, 1930). A patient educator's awareness of conditioning through external influence and the role that reinforcement plays in learning and behavior change can be valuable in patient teaching for lifestyle improvement. Behaviorism supports the position that positive or negative reinforcement can affect the patient's (pupil's) motivation, which can have direct consequences on the provision of healthcare and the establishment and implementation of a treatment plan. As discussed earlier, negative mental associations will need to be addressed. The patient may not want to follow up with the physician because of a negative mental association regarding physician visits. Explaining the purpose of future visits for the treatment plan may help alleviate the patient's fear.

Skinner tried to explain human language using behaviorism underpinnings (Overskeid, 1995). Chomsky challenged Skinner's behavioral position with the notion that individuals choose syntax in verbal communication (Chomsky, 1959; Green, 1994). Though the cognitive processes of attention, consciousness, memory, and perception are mentioned in behaviorist theory, behaviorism does not focus on the brain's inner functions (Cognitivism, 2009; Overskeid, 1995).

Cognitivism

Cognitivism is sometimes referred to as classical theory. In the 1950s and 1960s researchers began to investigate learning from inside the human brain, focusing on human thought. This new approach to thinking was called *cognitivism*—the science of the mind (Feldman & McPhee, 2008; Roland, 2008). Cognitivism posited that the human brain has more advanced abilities than the animal brain, and that the human brain is capable of higher-order processing of information (Roland, 2008). The capacity to apply logic and be rational in the processing of information is evidence of the higher-level function of the human brain (Ramey, 2005; Roland, 2008). The cognitivist view of the human brain is similar to how the central processing unit in a computer functions. They believe that information enters the brain, and then human thought processes the information (Feldman & McPhee, 2008).

Piaget's work in cognitive development and educational psychology made significant contributions to the theory of cognitivism. Piaget postulated that a person's interaction with the world played a role in the formation of mental concepts and a mental representation of reality (Piaget, 1954, 1967; Piotrowski, 2005). Piaget identified cognitive development in four stages: sensorimotor, preoperative, concrete operational, and formal operational (Piaget, 1954, 1967; Piotrowski, 2005; Santrock, 2007, 2008). Piaget deemed language a tool that contributes to cognitive development through exercises of personal interaction with the world (Piaget, 1954, 1967; Piotrowski, 2005; Santrock, 2008). He believed that language was directly reflective of cognitive maturity (Mayer, 1987; Piotrowski, 2005). Young children, because of immature and egocentric thought, are not concerned with external opinion. According to Piaget, with age and the mastery of logical thinking and perception, productive social interaction is achievable (Piaget, 1954, 1967; Piotrowski, 2005; Santrock, 2007, 2008). As people age they are able to focus beyond self and become more conscious of others (Piaget, 1954, 1967).

Cognitivists believe that learning involves mental associations (Ramey, 2005). Humans possess systematic internal capabilities that are used to elucidate their surroundings (Ramey, 2005). Information received is managed according to how it meaningfully corresponds with stored data called *schema* (Shuell, 1990). Schema theory, a subtheory of cognitivism developed by R.C. Anderson, postulates that schemata are mental representations that serve to network knowledge so it can be used by the mind (Anderson & Montauge, 1984; Davis, 1991). Schemata are used by the mind to govern behavior, organize memories, interpret information or experiences, and focus attention (Armbruster, 1996; Shuell, 1990). According to this theory, recall and understanding are contingent on how new information merges with existing established schema (Anderson & Montauge, 1984; Davis, 1991).

Cognitivists believe that variations in understanding, learning, and problem-solving capabilities among people are related to the variations in mental schemata (Shuell, 1990). Each individual's schema is unique because of varying personal experiences. The attachment of new information to present schema is meaning driven via personal interpretation (Armbruster, 1996). The schema theory can clarify the cognitive differences between a novice and an expert with regard to a skill (Shuell, 1990). A novice schema does not contain the wealth of specific topic information from which an expert can draw, who has expertise on that specific topic. Expert schemata contain a large and well-organized body of skill, knowledge, and experience that can be quickly accessed for use. This allows the expert to intervene and maneuver more quickly and with greater precision than a novice (Durso, Nickerson, Dumais, Lewandowsky, & Perfect, 2007). With time and practice, a novice may progress to an expert level (Durso et al., 2007).

It is imperative that educators help learners build schema and make mental connections by showing learners how the new information fits with previous connections (Balota, 2004). In healthcare, patients sometimes have difficulty understanding the rationale for self-care recommendations that they are advised to carry out. Helping the patient understand what is happening within their body provides a rationale for action that can bridge the connection to treatment options and ultimately help patients with their healthcare choices. Using an analogy, such as comparing the heart function to an engine or water pump, can help learners bridge new information with known information (Balota, 2004).

Stage theory, another subtheory of cognitivism, focuses on the human processing of information in three stages: (1) the input stage, (2) the short-term memory stage, and (3) the stage of information consolidation in long-term memory (Balota, 2004; Durso et al., 2007; Feldman & McPhee, 2008; Stuart-Hamilton, 2006). The input stage is where information is received and becomes internalized through encoding (Balota, 2004; Stuart-Hamilton, 2006). The dual encoding effect contends that memory contains two separate but interrelated systems—verbal and visual—for information processing (Feldman & McPhee, 2008).

In the second stage, information moves into the short-term memory, where it is retained for approximately 20 seconds unless it is rehearsed or grouped with meaningful information (Ross, 2006). The third and final stage includes the transition of information into long-term memory via rehearsal and or strong emotional context (Demetriou & Raftopoulos, 2005; Feldman & McPhee, 2008; Ross, 2006; Stuart-Hamilton, 2006). Short-term memory can only hold approximately seven units or pieces of information. After that volume is reached, the information is not retained because of short-term memory storage limitations and information over-load (Feldman & McPhee, 2008; Miller, 1956; Ross, 2006; Stuart-Hamilton, 2006). To compensate for the memory's limitations, Miller (1956) developed a method called *chunking*. In chunking, bits of information are loaded into cognitive chunks, which are constructed for easier transfer from short-term to long-term memory (Anderson & Montauge, 1984; Davis, 1991; Miller, 1956; Ross, 2006). This process of organizing information into chunks is known as the *cognitive load theory*, which is a subtheory of cognitivism.

Cognitivism is comprised of individual discoveries identified as principles that add significance to the teaching and learning process. One principle of cognitivism states that meaningful information is easier to learn and remember (Demetriou, & Raftopoulos, 2005; Feldman &

McPhee, 2008). People learn what is of interest to them (Knowles, 1972; Knowles, Holton, & Swanson, 2005). Another principle contends that the placement of information in presentation is relevant for memory. The serial position effect notes that items at the beginning or end of a list are easier to learn (Feldman & McPhee, 2008; Ross, 2006; Sousa, 2006). The distributed practice effect states that practice at intervals rather than all at one time is more effective (Demetriou, & Raftopoulos, 2005; Feldman & McPhee, 2008; Shuell, 1990). This principle is often used in sports. For example, consider a child who is learning how to play a sport. The child may show a natural aptitude for this sport. To ensure that the child is successful in the development and maintenance of their sport talent, they have to practice. Practice does not just happen once. Instead, practice will become a routine activity for the child. Rehearsal of the sport is a strategic exercise that gradually improves performance. As another example, consider a patient who has to begin a regimen of daily self-injections. At first, the patient may need step-by-step written instructions that can be followed while performing the injection. After multiple occurrences of self-injecting, the instructions will no longer be needed because the information and skill will have become ingrained in the memory. The practice of the skill will improve the knowledge and performance of the procedure.

The interference effect claims that prior learning can interfere with new learning if it is not filed correctly or is erroneous information (Anderson, & Speiro, 1977; Roediger & Karpicke, 2006). Interference effect often occurs when a person is given too much information to remember (Roediger & Karpicke, 2006). An example of interference effect is when a healthcare provider tells a patient four things they need to do, like taking their medication for infection twice a day with meals until the bottle is empty, losing weight, returning to the clinic in three or four weeks, and taking the chart to the window to pay. The likelihood of the patient forgetting one of the healthcare provider's recommendations is high. The information can become confused in encoding. Unfortunately, this is quite common since providers frequently give patients a lengthy list of things they are supposed to do for treatment. Continuing with the previous example, the physician tells a patient four things they need to do, and then the nurse lists an additional three things to do, followed by another list of two things from the pharmacist. It is easy to see how the multiple items can become confused. Planned previewing of information can have the opposite effect by enhancing memory. The effects of advanced organization affirm that previewing information and organizing that information into categories can reveal relationships that enhance learning (Feldman & McPhee, 2008; Sousa, 2006).

The theory of cognitivism provides some ideas about what could occur mentally in the teaching and learning process while offering educators some tactical considerations for information construction and delivery (Marr, 1971; Willshaw & Buckingham, 1990). With regard to learning, cognitivists do support the position that detailed, meaningful, clear, organized information is easier to understand, use, and apply (Demetriou & Raftopoulos, 2005; Feldman & McPhee, 2008; Sousa, 2006). Cognitivism also highlights some aspects of learning motivation and retention through identifying the power of meaningful information and the memory creation that occurs with interest or strong emotional ties to content (Demetriou & Raftopoulos, 2005; Feldman & McPhee, 2008; Knowles, 1968, 1972; Ross, 2006; Stuart-Hamilton, 2006). Cognitivism requires the educator to link information to the student. Information linking, according to cognitivism, may occur through the linking of new knowledge to known knowledge, through rehearsal and practice, or through mental connections accessed through emotional ties (Feldman & McPhee, 2008; Sousa, 2006).

Constructionism

Constructionism is a psychological theory of knowledge acquisition and is viewed as a core theory of learning. Constructionism asserts that learners construct knowledge and meaning from their experience, and that each learner individually defines new information using his experience. Constructionists see the mind as a creator of meaning. Constructionism contends that information can be imposed, but understanding is personal and can only come from within (Feldman & McPhee, 2008). This theory posits that the individual learner determines the significance of information through the convergence of self-knowledge and experience with new information (Lund, Carruth, Moody, & Logan, 2005; Saunders, 1992). According to constructionism, without the mental personalization of information, all information presented would simply accumulate in storage in the brain. When information is received, the learner merges new and previous information through mental processing or "construction" yielding a new representation (Lund et al., 2005; Saunders, 1992). The new mental representation or "construct" incorporates meaning intrinsic to the individual. The new "construct" possesses meaning, which embodies the learned information, through personal understanding. Constructionism captures the individualism of the learned experience inclusive of personal experience, previous knowledge, and the uniqueness of knowing (Brunner, 1990).

 ## Case Study

Dolly, an occupational therapist at the local hospital, and Kim, a teacher at the local high school, have both been diagnosed with breast cancer and both of their surgeons recommend total mastectomies. Dolly, as an occupational therapist, has cared for many patients who have had breast cancer. Dolly is familiar with several of the treatment options available and their success rates. Kim has lost a mother and sister to breast cancer. Neither Kim's mother nor Kim's sister had total mastectomies. Kim was present for all of the treatments her mother and sister went through. Although Dolly and Kim have the same diagnosis, their personal experiences and previous knowledge about the diagnosis are very different. Though the information provided about Dolly and Kim is only a snapshot of their different exposures and histories with breast cancer, it helps display immediate variance in personal influence. The personal influence from life and knowledge will ultimately have bearing on Dolly and Kim's construction of meaning for their diagnosis.

Penny, the social worker for the hospital, has been assigned to both Dolly's and Kim's cases. After listening to both of their histories including their exposure to breast cancer in their personal lives, Penny decides to offer both Dolly and Kim her contact information and a follow-up visit for the following week. Dolly states that she does not want to wait; she will be having her surgery next week and would like to know what she needs to do now. Kim, on the other hand, tells Penny that she appreciates her time and she will see her next week at her scheduled appointment. Both patients have the same diagnosis, but both patients are at different points in their processing of the information and decisions to act. Penny allowed both patients the autonomy to freely move at their own pace.

Expert Support for Action

Fear, lack of control, and grieving for loss of health are all emotions that patients are likely to experience in healthcare (Jervey, 2001; Mitchell, Murray, & Hynson, 2008). Kübler-Ross identified five stages of grief that are commonly seen in persons who experience loss (Kübler-Ross, 1969). Losses ranging from the death of a loved one to the loss of a job can trigger the grief process. The five stages of Kübler-Ross's grief cycle include (1) denial, (2) anger, (3) bargaining, (4) depression, and (5) acceptance. Kübler-Ross described grief as an individual process, while Hamilton noted the fluidity and nonlinear nature of the grieving process (Hamilton, 2005; Kübler-Ross & Kessler, 2005). The entire decision process is influenced by the patient's health status and other influences like physical, mental, financial, environmental, social, culture, and spiritual beliefs (Falvo, 1994; Henderson, 2002; Pierce & Hicks, 2001; Prossier, Almond, & Walley, 2003; Stewart, Meredith, Brown, & Galajda, 2000).

Piaget's work in the identification of mechanisms used in the process of internalizing knowledge serves as the core of the theory of constructionism. According to Piaget, new knowledge is constructed through the processes of accommodation and assimilation (Ausubel et al., 1986; Lund et al., 2005; Novak, 1998; Saunders, 1992). Accommodation is the process where reframing of the mental representation occurs to accommodate the inclusion of new information (Atherton 2009). Accommodation is a more advanced process than assimilation, which involves the rearranging of present knowledge (Feldman & McPhee, 2008). Previous knowledge is altered to allow for the inclusion of newly acquired information. Accommodation requires learner effort in mental processing, cognitive storage, and practice (Ormrod, 2008).

Conversely, in assimilation, the new information joins into an existing cognitive framework without changing that framework (Ausubel et al., 1986; Lund et al., 2005; Novak, 1998; Saunders, 1992). The assimilation process is relatively passive because the new information is similar and easy to associate with previously embedded information. Although Piaget's work was paramount to constructionism theory, Jerome Bruner first introduced the concept of learning as knowledge-building or construction (Bruner, 1990; Feldman & McPhee, 2008). Bruner built on the work of Lev Vygotsky, a Soviet psychologist who introduced scaffolding as a method of teaching in education (Ausubel et al., 1986; Feldman & McPhee, 2008; Saunders, 1992). Scaffolding is a method by which the instructor provides support and guidance for students as they transition to a higher level of thinking or skill (Ausubel et al., 1986; Feldman &

McPhee, 2008; Saunders, 1992; Sthapornnanon et al., 2009). Once the skill is mastered, then fading, or the gradual removal of support, occurs leaving the student to successfully function independently (Lipscomb, Swanson, & West, 2004; Sthapornnanon et al., 2009).

Because constructionism highlights the personalization of the learning experience, an active learner is needed for successful learning (Ausubel et al., 1986; Saunders, 1992). The teaching methods of constructionism use problem solving, thinking strategies, discussion, and real world situations to teach learners (Mayer, 1987; Sthapornnanon et al., 2009). Learning heightens in situations that help link information through active knowing and doing (Mayer, 1987; Sthapornnanon et al., 2009). These situations may be real world, simulation, or case study. Whatever the context, the learning situation requires the learner to solve problems and build upon existing knowledge. The teacher stimulates thinking by asking questions and offering feedback, but the student is encouraged to resolve the situation via personal conclusions (Meek, 2009; Mayer, 1987; Sthapornnanon et al., 2009).

 ## Case Study

After teaching Mr. Johnston, the president of the local bank, about his Coumadin medication, his patient educator Nancy started asking Mr. Johnson how he would respond if he noticed blood in his stool or urine. Nancy did not provide Mr. Johnston with the answer. Instead, she listened as Mr. Johnston walked Nancy through exactly what he would do, step by step. Nancy provides feedback and guidance, but Mr. Johnston had to move the passive information into an action state.

Expert Support for Action

Redman (2007) asserts that patients need a rationale for ordered treatment, especially when behavior change is involved. Bloom's original taxonomy moved from the lowest level of thought—knowledge through comprehension, application, analysis, and synthesis—to evaluation, the highest level (Bloom, 1956). As the student moves from knowledge toward evaluation, their ability to comprehend and utilize information becomes more complex. The progression of Bloom's taxonomy follows the student's transition from familiarity to ownership and, finally, mastery of information. The capacity to apply logic and be rational in the processing of information exposes more of the higher-level function of the human brain (Ramey, 2005; Roland, 2008). Immediate use of learned information can boost the retention rate up to 90% (Ormrod, 2008; Sousa, 2006).

Two general frameworks that can be used to create a constructionist learning environment are outlined in the following lists (Feldman & McPhee, 2008).

The first is Bybee's 5-E framework: Engage, Explore, Explain, Elaborate, and Evaluate (Bybee, 1966; Lord, 1997).

1. Engage: Find out the extent of student knowledge about a topic, what needs to be known, and then stimulate the student's interest to know more.

2. Explore: Allow the student to get involved with the learning materials and let them share what they are thinking, observing, and experiencing.

3. Explain: Provide opportunity for the student to make sense of his discoveries and analysis. Allow the student to identify and interpret while providing correct information as the facilitator of the experience so that the information learned is accurate.

4. Elaborate: Allow the student to use understanding of the concepts in new situations while comparing his previous experiences with his new ones.

5. Evaluate: At every stage of the model, provide feedback and direction while ensuring correct understanding is being achieved.

The second framework is the learning cycle, which uses a three-step design:

1. Discovery: The teacher allows the student to generate questions and hypotheses from working with various sources.

2. Concept introduction: The teacher works with the student to help him work through questions, hypotheses, and experimentation designed to stimulate understanding.

3. Concept application: The student moves the problem into new situations in a quest for resolution and greater understanding.

In summary, constructionism focuses on strategically building knowledge by gradually adding new knowledge to old knowledge while incrementally moving the student to a higher level of knowing. The educator focuses on ensuring proper placement of new knowledge so that the appropriate connections are made, resulting in solid construction. Constructionism helps the educator understand the importance of a discovery and exploration safe zone, so the student can sample real world experiences without real life consequences. The educator selects projects that can advance the student's knowledge base. A constructionist educator's intent is for the student to safely be able to explore new information under supervision and guidance. The educator serves to facilitate the students' mental connections while supporting their mental connections.

Each of the three learning theories views the process of learning differently. Figure 5-3 displays each theory and its philosophy toward the

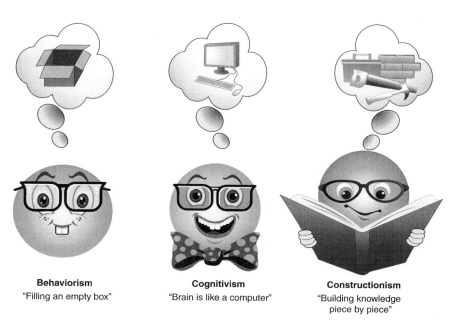

Behaviorism	Cognitivism	Constructionism
"Filling an empty box"	"Brain is like a computer"	"Building knowledge piece by piece"

Figure 5-3. Three theoretical learning perspectives are depicted to illustrate different theoretical views of learning. Behaviorism asserts that learning is like filling an empty box. Cognitivism views the brain as a computer or central processor in learning. Constructionism views knowledge as building or construction, adding a piece of information at a time.

learning process. All three theories offer viewpoints that can assist patient educators as they teach patients. Seeing each patient interaction as an opportunity to add knowledge correlates with the behaviorist view that each pupil's mind in learning is like a box being filled. Recognizing the receiver's mind as a computer that processes information, as with a cognitivist view, helps an educator remember to honor the student's need for time to internally process information. Borrowing the constructionist perspective of learning can help an educator remember to thoughtfully place information for the construction of solid and lasting knowledge. Each theory can enhance the art of patient education.

SUMMARY

- For learning to occur, information has to have logical order for the brain to be able to receive, process, and ultimately store the information.

- Planning and preparing patient information, just as a teacher plans and prepares student information, offers an opportunity for healthcare providers to capitalize on proven academic techniques that can improve the possibility that the receiver—the patient—is successful in understanding the information delivered.

- Packaging information for delivery can present a challenge for educators, especially in healthcare.

- Many times, one-on-one teaching sessions are at the convenience of the educator and do not coincide with optimal timing for the patient.

- Scheduled one-on-one teaching sessions can allow the patient to add input to the direction of the teaching interaction. Educators must be open and encourage patients to identify and share their self-diagnosed knowledge needs.

- Engaging a learner involves a concerted physical effort to show the learner that they are your present focus.

- In constructing and planning what information needs to be delivered, knowing the patient's level of knowledge on a topic is beneficial.

- In the 1950s, Benjamin Bloom identified learning domains that include six levels of human thought that differ in complexity.

- Bloom organized his cognitive levels into a taxonomy that many educators use in the construction of educational learning goals and objectives.

- In the teaching of patients, understanding the levels of knowledge can help the patient educator in moving the patient from a level of *remember* to *apply*.

- Teaching and learning are intensely personal activities; not all teachers are the same and, more importantly, not all learners are the same.

- Knowing a person's learning style can help the educator tailor the delivery of information to the learner's preferred (and most effective) learning style.

- There are three types of perceptual processing learning styles: visual, tactile, and auditory.

- Material delivered according to a personal learning style can help the learner receive and process the information with ease, while increasing the likelihood for overall success in the learner's educational experience.

- In learning, knowledge or an understanding is gained by study, instruction, or experience. Learning is a science.

- Three prominent theoretical views hold sway in education regarding how learning occurs and factors that influence learning: behaviorism, cognitivism, and constructionism. These theories are considered influences of medagogy.

- Behaviorists define learning as a change in behavior due to experience and the creation of habits. They see the mind metaphorically as an empty container. Behaviorists believe that human learning can only be explained through observable behaviors.

- Implications for the practice of patient education derived from the behaviorism theory center around a belief that knowledge is not something that exists in the mind, but instead works as a form of guidance formed from actions.

- The cognitivist view of the human brain is similar to how the central processing unit in a computer functions. They believe that information enters the brain, and then human thought processes the information.

- Cognitivists believe that learning involves mental associations. Humans possess systematic internal capabilities that are used to elucidate their surroundings. Information received is managed according to how it meaningfully corresponds with stored data called *schema*.

- Cognitivism highlights some aspects of learning motivation and retention through identifying the power of meaningful information in learning and the memory creation that occurs with interest or strong emotional ties to content.

- Constructionism asserts that learners construct knowledge and meaning based on their experience, and that each learner individually defines new information using their experience. Constructionists see the mind as a creator of meaning.

- Constructionism focuses on strategically building knowledge by gradually adding new knowledge to old knowledge while incrementally moving the student to a higher level of knowing.

- All three theories offer viewpoints that can serve patient educators as they teach patients. Each theory can enhance the art of patient education.

[CHAPTER 6]

Health Promotion Theories

Since patient education is central to healthcare, it can behoove the healthcare provider to be aware of existing health promotion theories. To better understand the relationship that health plays in a patient's acquisition of knowledge, three popular health theories will be reviewed briefly: the health belief model, the PRECEDE-PROCEED health education planning model, and the health promotion model.

HEALTH BELIEF MODEL

In the mid-1950s, when public health started to move toward preventive care, a group of researchers at the U. S. Public Health Service developed the health belief model (Green, 2002; Kirscht, Haefner, Kegeles, & Rosenstock, 1966; Rosenstock, 1966). The model explained and predicted health behaviors stemming from a person's beliefs about the health problem and the health behavior. In the mid-1970s, Marshall Becker updated the model by adding measurement scales. The health belief model remained in vogue as the most used theoretical framework in health education until the early 1990s (Green, 2002).

The model contains four basic elements: (1) belief in personal susceptibility, (2) perception of severity, (3) personal benefit, and (4) cues to action (Davies, 2006; Green, 2002; Rosenstock, Strecher, & Becker, 1988). If a person feels that there is significant personal risk for a health problem, he may consider action. If the personal benefit of action outweighs the perceived barriers to action, then action toward change may be considered.

If the person feels that he could successfully perform the new action, then action is more likely to occur (Davies, 2006; Green, 2002; Redman, 2001; Rosenstock, 1966; Rosenstock, Strecher, & Becker, 1988).

The health belief model successfully explores the personal impetus for health behavior and provides a unique insight into patient focus as a change in health behavior is contemplated. Although the model was developed to predict the adoption or rejection of healthy behavior, it has been argued that it is more successful at helping providers understand the cessation of unhealthy behavior (McIntosh & Kubena, 1996; Rosenstock, Strecher, & Becker, 1988). The model is based on two variables: the psychological state of preparedness and the belief that action is needed and will be helpful (Rosenstock, 1966). Becker (1974) asserts that empirical data reveals the impact a healthcare provider's personal involvement can have on gaining patient attention and solidifying patient understanding. Understanding the relationship between patients' perceptions and the elements that influence their choices to move toward action can empower healthcare providers as they communicate health information to their patients. Consider a patient who is at risk for diabetes because of family history, compared with a patient who has diabetes and is suffering from signs and symptoms. The at-risk patient may not be ready for behavior changes because no diabetes-related ill effects are experienced, whereas the patient that is experiencing ill effects related to the diagnosis may have a stronger belief that behavior changes are needed.

  Case Study

Leah is a 22-year-old college student. Since Leah enrolled at the local community college she has assumed a more sedentary lifestyle inclusive of fast food and sugar consumption. During her annual exam her healthcare provider, Jana, noted the change in Leah's lifestyle and her strong maternal family history of adult-onset diabetes. Leah's weight has consistently increased by 8 to 10 pounds annually. Jana began to discuss her risk of diabetes during the visit. Leah gathered her belongings as her provider spoke but offered no sign that she was listening and no acknowledgement of reception or understanding. After the visit Leah's mother asked Leah how her appointment went. Without hesitation, Leah responded "fine." The concept of diabetes had no impact on Leah because she could not relate to what the provider was discussing. Because she has exhibited no symptoms or complications from diabetes, the diagnosis did not belong to her and was therefore deemed to not be relevant to her life. The significance of sedentary lifestyle and weight gain did not correlate with the prospective change in health related to diabetes.

The next day Jana called Leah to give her the results from some lab work Leah had drawn on her visit. Jana told Leah that her blood glucose was elevated and she wanted her to have more lab work done. Leah told Jana that she had eaten candy just before the blood work was done and that she did not think it was necessary to do more blood work when the values weren't really that bad. Jana started to tell Leah about the damage that diabetes can cause in the body when she was interrupted by Leah, who informed Jana that her mother has diabetes and she knows all about the disease. Jana asked Leah if she would indulge her and come to a free meeting at the hospital at 7 PM. Leah asked why. Jana said she felt that Leah may be able to get something out of the meeting while helping others. Leah agreed and showed up for the meeting. Jana facilitated the meeting, which was a support group for the families of diabetic patients. Leah was frustrated at first when she found out what the meeting was for but as she listened to the participants she began to connect with their messages. Discussions of risks and fears, as well as frustrations, filled the hour. Before she knew it Jana was thanking everyone for their participation and reminding them of the scheduled time for their next meeting. After the meeting Leah approached Jana to find out where she needed to go for her lab work.

Expert Support for Action

Emotions can be a significant challenge to patient learning (Dube, Belanger, & Trudeau, 1996; Ong, Visser, Lammes, & de Haes, 2000). Malcolm Knowles (1950) proposes that as individuals mature into adults, their concepts of self change the manner in which they approach learning. In andragogic methodology, the instructor shifts from the pedagogic role of source of information to the facilitator role of expert resource who helps guide the learner toward knowledge (Knowles et al., 2005). In andragogy, the learner is self-directed, actively seeking and moving toward knowledge. The employment of various resources and methodologies assist the instructor in guiding the learner toward desired information (Knowles, 1950, 1975).

PRECEDE-PROCEED HEALTH EDUCATION PLANNING MODEL

In 1980, Green and colleagues published the PRECEDE framework for health education planning. PRECEDE is an acronym for **P**redisposing, **R**einforcing, and **E**nabling **C**auses in **E**ducational **D**iagnosis and **E**valuation. The model consists of seven stages to be used in the planning of health education. In 1991, Green and Kreuter revisited the PRECEDE framework and transitioned the model into the more useful PRECEDE-PROCEED planning model.

PROCEED is an acronym for **P**olicy, **R**egulatory, and **O**rganizational **C**onstructs in **E**ducational and **E**nvironmental **D**evelopment. PRECEDE provides a problem-solving strategy to support the planning of specific and intentional health education programs. PROCEED complements programs that are designed using PRECEDE by providing structured guidance through implementation and evaluation of these programs (Green & Mercer, 2009).

Historically, the PRECEDE-PROCEED model has been used to organize and provide direction for the development of health programs. The model is used to plan and organize activities over time to meet certain health-related goals (Green & Kreuter, 2005). PRECEDE consists of five stages that are followed by four stages of PROCEED. The PRECEDE stages are (1) social assessment and situational analysis, (2) epidemiologic assessment, (3) behavioral and environmental assessment, (4) educational and organizational assessment, (5) administrative and policy assessment. PROCEED consists of (6) intervention implementation, (7) process evaluation, (8) impact evaluation, and (9) outcome evaluation (Green & Kreuter, 2005). Each of the nine stages has a specific focus for users to concentrate on as they progress in planning, implementation, and finally, evaluation (Cannick et al., 2007). The PRECEDE-PROCEED model is intended to flow in an uninterrupted cycle with PROCEED stages to follow immediately after the PRECEDE stages (Green & Mercer, 2003). The flow of the model guides the user's perspective from broad to detailed in implementation, then from detailed to broad in evaluation.

Each stage's area of concentration helps move the user from a universal overarching intent to an action, which is implemented and evaluated as the user moves back through each stage to the original universal overarching intent. The flow of PRECEDE-PROCEED offers a solid and logical platform on which to build a public health education program. However, individual education is not the focus of the PRECEDE-PROCEED model. This model is commonly used to strategically plan for community courses related to specific diagnosis or prevention programs.

HEALTH PROMOTION MODEL

The health promotion model (HPM) created by Nola Pender was first published in 1982. Pender's model is based on two theories: social cognitive theory and expectancy value theory. The psychologist Albert Bandura's social cognitive theory focused on personal self-confidence related to action and explained human behavior as constant interaction of cognitive, behavioral, and environmental influences (Bandura, 1977). The psychologist Martin Fishbein's expectancy value theory postulates that people are more likely to participate in activity they feel is valuable and achievable (Fishbein, 1963). Pender revised her model in 1996 to increase explanatory power and the model's use in creating health-promoting actions (Peterson & Bredow, 2009).

Pender's model strongly supports the partner relationship between provider and healthcare consumer. The HPM serves to provide an understanding of the process people participate in when choosing whether to engage in health-promoting behaviors (Pender, Murdaugh, & Parsons, 2002). The HPM first connects the consumer's individual choices to specific competing preferences and demands to commitment, and then to behaviors.

Pender, Murdaugh, and Parsons (2002) acknowledge that there are seven assumptions for Pender's HPM model. These assumptions are:

- Individuals desire an environment in which they can achieve their unique health potential.
- Individuals possess ability for reflective self-awareness and self-assessment of personal competencies.
- Individuals' value grows in a positive direction as they strive to achieve a balance between change and stability.
- People seek to control their own behavior.
- People interact with their environment, and because of this they are changed and the environment is changed.

- Healthcare professionals are a part of the environment and have influence on people throughout the lifespan.

- Ultimate control is with self; self-initiated alteration of the person-environment relationship is necessary for behavior change.

There are 11 concepts in Pender's HPM. The first concept, personal factors (biological, psychological, and sociocultural), are those associated with the person and influence health-promoting activity (e.g., race, physical activity, and family) (Peterson & Bredow, 2009). The next concept, prior related behaviors, refers to an individual's previous exposure to the health-promoting behavior. Behavior-specific cognitions and affect have six concepts: perceived benefits of action, perceived barriers to action, perceived self-efficacy, activity-related affect, interpersonal influences, and situational influences (Pender, Murdaugh, & Parsons, 2002). Behavioral outcomes, the final category, has three concepts: immediate competing demands and preferences, commitment to a plan of action, and health-promoting behavior (Pender, Murdaugh, & Parsons, 2002).

Pender's model helps to identify the influences involved in personal movement toward healthy behavior. Understanding the multifaceted nature of people as they move toward health, including their interpersonal relationships and physical environments, can assist patient educators and healthcare providers in understanding patients and their individual challenges.

OTHER CHANGE THEORIES RELEVANT TO PATIENT EDUCATORS

The following change theories will be discussed briefly: theory of reasoned action, theory of planned behavior, self-management theory, self-leadership theory, self-efficacy theory, interpersonal theory, social networking theory, and transtheoretical theory. Healthcare treatment usually requires a patient to change his behavior. These behavior-change theories can offer insight into the concepts, relationships, and influences that occur when a patient is contemplating change.

Theories of Reasoned Action and Planned Behavior

The theory of reasoned action (TRA), a predictive persuasion theory, was introduced in 1975 by two social psychologists, Ajzen and Fishbein.

According to this model, personal beliefs and bias directly influence a person's attitude toward a behavior, which in turn directly impacts his behavioral intention and ultimately his actual behavior (Fishbein & Ajzen, 1975). The three main concepts of TRA are behavioral intention (BI), attitudes (A), and subjective norms (SN) (Fishbein & Ajzen, 1975).

TRA maintains that behavioral intention is the sum of personal attitudes and subjective norms: $BI = A + SN$. According to TRA, attitudes are individual beliefs about a behavior, and subjective norms are an individual's beliefs in a social environment. TRA suggests that a person's individual and social group beliefs can ultimately impact behavior (Fishbein & Ajzen, 1975). This theory highlights not only the role personal value plays in the execution of a behavior, but also the importance external approval, such as family and peer approval, can have on behavior (Ajzen & Fishbein, 1980). TRA serves to provide a conceptual framework defining links between attitudes, social norms, and individual behavior (Ajzen, & Fishbein, 1980).

In 1985, after the TRA theory was included in a relevant study, Ajzen discovered that behavior was not completely voluntary as previously supposed in TRA. Ajzen added control beliefs and perceived behavioral beliefs as major variables to the TRA model and named his new model the theory of planned behavior (TPB) (Ajzen, 2006). TPB helps predict deliberate and planned behavior including actual behavioral control as an influence on a person's behavior.

Social Influence and Personal Management Theories

Interpersonal theory and social networking theory are similar in that they focus on the influence other people can have on an individual's actions. Social networking theory proposes that networks of relationships help shape individuals, their beliefs, and ultimately their behavior (Hill & Dunbar, 2002). Interpersonal theory focuses on the social aspect of humans and relationships. Interpersonal theory relates how present and past personal interactions shape personal choice and action (Sullivan, 2003). Both of these theories are concentrated on the role of social influences in personal behavior. Awareness of these theoretical perspectives can assist the patient educator in holistically planning a patient's educational regimen.

Self-management theory concentrates on empowering a person to control a behavior (Redman, 2001). In self-management, the use of self-awareness, personal monitoring of internal cues, and use of external cues for healthy alternative behavior enable individuals to take control and manage their personal health-behavior choices. This independence allows a person to progress toward personal health goals.

Self-leadership theory, like self-management theory, focuses on personal empowerment. In self-leadership theory, personal empowerment can serve as a motivational construct that establishes opportunity through which persons can articulate themselves to a level of improved capabilities and performance (Bandura, 1994).

Bandura's self-efficacy theory (Bandura, 1997) concentrates on individuals' self-perceived capabilities to control their behavior and circumstances in their lives (Bandura, 1994). In self-efficacy theory, a person's perspective on their capabilities influences how they view their potential for success when facing challenges. A person with high self-efficacy maintains a sense of personal ability to accomplish. This type of person embraces difficult situations with a desire to master or conquer. In contrast, individuals with low self-efficacy are filled with doubt and tend to give up easily when facing challenges. During difficult circumstances, those with high self-efficacy focus on ways to succeed, while those with low self-efficacy focus on personal deficits and lack of ability. In Bandura's theory, personal feelings about self-ability, positive or negative, progress beyond the affective realm into the behavioral realm (Bandura, 1994). Self-efficacy theory postulates that personal feeling regarding self-ability influences self-motivation and, ultimately, behavior (Bandura, 1997).

Progress Toward Change Theories

The transtheoretical model (TTM) focuses on identifying where a person is regarding personal decision-making and commitment to a behavior-changing action (Prochaska, 2009). Transtheoretical theory is composed of six stages: precontemplation, contemplation, preparation, action, maintenance, and termination (Prochaska & Velicer, 1997; Spring, 2008). Each stage of transtheoretical theory is defined according to its proximity to actual behavior change (Prochaska, 2009).

Motivational interviewing is a counseling technique often used in health coaching to encourage a person to move through the stages of behavior change (Miller & Rollnick, 2002). Figure 6-1 depicts the inclusion of these theories as a patient tries to make healthcare decisions in the progression toward behavior change or action. Understanding the mental progression that must occur to bring about action for behavior change can help identify how close the person is to implementing a new behavior.

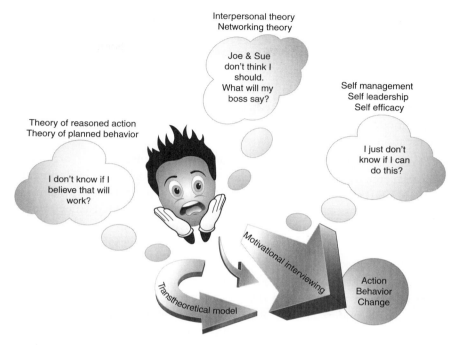

Figure 6-1. This illustration displays choice and action theories represented in thoughts that might occur in the decision-making process. The thoughts move from one's own ability, the opinions of one's social network, and the effectiveness of the proposed action toward proximity to action.

This knowledge can help the patient educator determine what information the patient will need to know and what skills must be mastered for safety and success.

SUMMARY

- Since patient education is central to health care, it behooves the health-care provider to be aware of existing health promotion theories.
- The health belief model explains and predicts health behaviors stemming from a person's beliefs about the health problem and the health behavior.

- The health belief model successfully explores the personal impetus for health behavior and provides a unique insight into patient focus as a change in health behavior is contemplated.

- In 1980, Green and colleagues published the PRECEDE framework for health education planning. PRECEDE is an acronym for predisposing, reinforcing, and enabling causes in educational diagnosis and evaluation. The model consists of seven stages to be used in the planning of health education.

- The PROCEED acronym stands for policy, regulatory, and organizational constructs in educational and environmental development. PRECEDE provides a problem-solving strategy to support the planning of intentional specific health education programs. PROCEED complements programs that are designed using PRECEDE by providing structured guidance through implementation and evaluation of these programs.

- Pender's health promotion model strongly supports the partner relationship between provider and healthcare consumer. The HPM serves to provide an understanding of the process people participate in when choosing whether to engage in health-promoting behaviors.

- According to the theory of reasoned action, personal beliefs and bias directly influence a person's attitude toward a behavior, which in turn directly impacts that person's behavioral intention and ultimately his actual behavior.

- Social networking theory proposes that networks of relationships help shape individuals, their beliefs, and ultimately their behavior.

- Interpersonal theory focuses on the social aspect of humans and relationships.

- In self-management theory, the use of self-awareness, personal monitoring of internal cues, and use of external cues for healthy alternative behavior enables people to take control and manage their health behavior choices. This independence enables progress toward personal health goals.

- In self-leadership theory, personal empowerment can serve as a motivational construct that establishes opportunity through which persons can articulate themselves to a level of improved capabilities and performance.

- Bandura's self-efficacy theory concentrates on individuals' self-perceived capabilities to control their behavior and circumstances in their lives.
- Transtheoretical model (TTM) focuses on identifying where a person is at regarding personal decision making and commitment to a behavior-changing action. Transtheoretical theory is composed of six stages: precontemplation, contemplation, preparation, action, maintenance, and termination.

SECTION II SUMMARY

Healthcare practice offers practitioners the challenge of teaching individuals who often unwittingly assume the role of student. These healthcare students may be patients or patients' significant others. Most often, the patients do not even realize they are students and are expected to assimilate all information that is given while a health crisis is transpiring. Too often the patients and their significant others are so overwhelmed with the emotional component of healthcare that they are unable to sustain the inherent learning component.

Although academically held principles of teaching can be replicated in healthcare, the student in the patient role is unique and varies greatly from the traditional academic student. For the healthcare student, the stakes involved with knowledge attainment and learning can be more serious. For the traditional classroom student, the greatest risk is receiving a poor letter grade or course failure. Failure for the healthcare pupil can mean loss of quality of life, independence, and even death. Information for the healthcare pupil can be life sustaining, and understanding is critical for successful outcomes.

Although a theory may originate in one discipline, the theory's implementation and utilization is limited only by the beholder. Theory provides definition to concepts with relational statements in a conceptual framework. The value of the theory lies in utilization and application. Theories can be reframed to fit the area of intended application, and provide patient educators with a foundational understanding and framework for use in their practice of patient education.

SECTION III

PATIENT KNOWLEDGE

[CHAPTER 7]

Patient Learning

In this section, the concept of patient information is reviewed. First, a quick overview focuses on the uniqueness of patient learning in healthcare. Then, a brief review of shared knowledge (discussed in detail in Chapter 1) transitions into an overview of how to move the patient from learning to knowing. An introduction to the concepts of evolution of patient information, patient educational hierarchy, and informational seasons of patient education adds structure to the discussion of patient education.

PATIENT LEARNING IN HEALTHCARE

Aristotle, in his first book of *Metaphysics*, asserted that the main difference between master craftsmen and manual workers lies in the former's grasp of the theory underlying their work (Aristole, 2009). Aristotle posits that within the understanding of "why" lies reason, which provides an insight or wisdom that can be used beyond the immediate intended utility. The wisdom Aristotle referred to empowers the master craftsman with an ability to influence beyond original intent to unforeseen possibilities of application. Put another way, the application of knowledge is limited only by the wisdom of the beholder.

Healthcare providers educate patients every day. Educators of patients usually borrow individual pieces and parts of facts from various sources with no consistency or personal knowledge of the reliability and effectiveness of the source (Brunetti & Hermes-DeSantis, 2010; Hesse et al., 2005; IOM, 2002). Inconsistency and oversight in the duties of patient education, as well as haphazard planning and delivery of patient information, are common to healthcare (Boyde et al., 2009; Close, 1988). Patients are taught daily in formal, planned sessions, as well as through informal, spontaneous interactions. A Swedish study found that although healthcare providers documented the act of educating patients, the actual patient education was "fragmented and vague" (Friberg, Bergh, & Lepp, 2006, p. 1551). The art and science of the practice of educating patients has consisted of providers finding a fit, mode, and method of information delivery that tended to worked best for themselves (Towle & Godolphin, 1999). Many times the act of educating patients is confused with basic exposure to information. Good patient education involves skillful construction undertaken so that delivered information can be understood, processed, remembered, and translated into self-care (Rogers, Wallace, & Weiss, 2006).

Experts argue that unskilled communication efforts of healthcare providers is to blame for their poor performance in patient education (Hoving, Visser, Mullen, van den Borne, 2010; Sandars & Esmail, 2003; Syred, 1981). Schwartzenburg and colleagues assert that healthcare professionals need to be trained in how to teach (Schwartzenberg, 2007). Poor patient-provider communication has been linked to a range of negative occurrences in health care, from poor health literacy to increased medical errors (Close, 1988; Sandars & Esmail, 2003). Excuses aside, the multibillion dollar annual price tag resulting from poor health literacy, as discussed in Chapter 1, validates the need to move toward definition and organization of patient education among all healthcare disciplines.

While the profession of academic education provides educational theories and conceptual frameworks for teaching and learning, there are unique and various circumstances that create obstacles on the road to understanding when the student is a patient, a receiver of healthcare services (Best, 2001; Gessner, 1989; Kick, 1989). Unfortunately, the learners found in typical educational theories and models are not equivalent to patient-students, and neither is the setting, the stakes, nor the message. Basically, only the goal of knowledge-transfer is shared (Veldtman et al., 2001). The uniqueness of the patient as a student creates the need to look at patient education as a special form of education, separate from traditionally held ideas about mainstream education that primarily occurs in academic institutions. Much like the educational awakening that occurred with the founding of andragogy, so is the much overdue need to differentiate the uniqueness of patient education from traditional education.

Healthcare naturally presents many obstacles for teaching and learning (Behar-Horenstein et al., 2005; Palazzo, 2009). Of course, any environment can pose barriers to learning. When learners have to overcome learning barriers, they have increased risk of making inappropriate assumptions, which can lead to error (Rogers, Wallace, & Weiss, 2006). In the healthcare setting, learning barriers may be personal, relational, cultural, structural, and societal (Iacono & Campbell, 1997; Spath, 2008; Veldtman et al., 2001). Personal learning barriers can include emotional and cognitive constraints as well as limitations related to values and beliefs (Gerteis, Edgman-Levitan, Daley, & Delbanco, 1993). Relational learning barriers may include issues in the history and background of the provider-patient relationship, caregiver-patient relationship, and physical disharmony that is unspoken but often communicated through body language (Anderson, Rainey, & Eysenbach, 2004; Roter, 1977). Others barriers may include variance in the provider's and patient's cultures including educational or learning backgrounds (Falvo, 1994; Galanti, 2008; Institute of Medicine of the National Academies, 2009). Structural barriers may include physical setting or teaching-learning environment (Lorig, 1992). Societal barriers include regulatory mandates, credentialing requirements, and professional standards regarding patient education (Falvo, 1994; Stewart, 2008). Societal barriers also include assumed structures differentiating separate roles, classes, rights, and privileges, as well as organizational values and financial constraints or incentives, productivity requirements, and time valuation or constraints (Galanti, 2008; Roter, 1977; Wlodkowski, 2008).

MOVING TOWARD SHARED KNOWLEDGE

In the healthcare setting, licensed healthcare providers serve as authorities on health, healthcare, disease, and treatment (Roter, 1977; Towle & Godolphin, 1999). While the licensed healthcare provider serves as a subject matter expert in health, the patient is an expert of self. Patients are uniquely positioned to possess full understanding of their personal lives, feelings, and all that has consciously been experienced by the self (Brodenheimer, Lorig, Holman, & Grumbach, 2002; Funnell & Anderson, 2004). Both experts, patient and provider, have influence, power, and

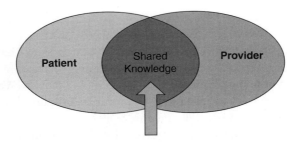

Figure 7-1. To build a foundation for partnership on which to plan care and build understanding, patient-provider knowledge should be merged.

ability to reach successful outcomes in their respective expertise (Towle & Godolphin, 1999; Wingate, 1990). The key to being successful lies in the effectiveness of patient-provider communication (Institute of Medicine of the National Academies, 2009).

Information needs to be openly exchanged in the provider-patient relationship. Information withheld from either party could directly impact potential outcomes. All information exchanged needs to be received and valued. Receiving information goes beyond simply hearing it. Receiving means the information is actually comprehended. Valued means the information has importance and worth. Both the patient and provider should receive and value the information provided and then merge it with personal expertise. The union of new information with personal expertise is used to provide a foundation of understanding that serves as shared knowledge for both parties to use in decision making in the patient-provider encounter (Figure 7-1).

The healthcare decision cycle (Figure 7-2) offers a visual of the impact and flow of information between experts, health expert and self expert, in the provider-patient relationship. Two conceptual streams are depicted in the healthcare decision cycle: information and choice. The information stream is composed of communicating and listening, which openly flows between provider and patient. Choice also streams openly between provider and patient. Choice and information run alongside each other, intersecting just prior to the reception of each party. Information and choice intersect at both the patient and provider levels, symbolizing the connection or influence each has with the other. The healthcare decision cycle visually displays how information is exchanged between the provider and patient, while simultaneously choices are arising between the provider and patient.

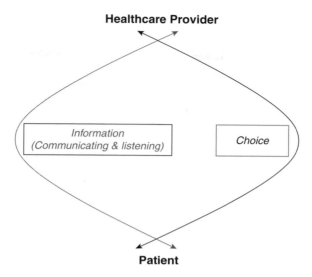

Figure 7-2. The healthcare decision cycle displays a constant flow of information between the provider and the patient (Stewart, 2009). Choice is noted as a constant exchange between the patient and provider. The two constants represented, information and choice, intersect on both the provider and patient ends to symbolize the influence both bear on the other. Choice is influenced by information, and information is influenced by choice.

FROM LEARNING TO KNOWING

All men by nature desire knowledge.

—Aristotle (384 BC–322 BC)

Trying to learn can be challenging for people even when they have identified a need for knowledge and are willing and ready to learn. The learning environment in healthcare is often complicated by factors that patients experience such as illness, emotions (e.g., fear, anger, insecurity, and sorrow), financial insult, pain, chaos, and urgency; it is easy to see how learning can become very challenging (Levinson, Gorawara-Bhat, & Lamb, 2000; Rolls, Horrak, Wade, & McGrath, 1994). While these factors may be encountered in a traditional academic setting, they are not common to every single student. In the healthcare environment, it is rare when these emotions are not present in patients (Clark, Drain, & Malone, 2003;

Gustafson, Arora, Nelson, & Boberg, 2003). Emotions, especially the negative and undesirable, can cause senses to heighten and interfere with information reception and processing in patient education (Dube, Belanger, & Trudeau, 1996; Ong, Visser, Lammess & de Haes, 2000).

Fear, lack of control, and grieving for loss of health are all emotions that patients are likely to experience in healthcare (Jervey, 2001; Mitchell, Murray, & Hynson, 2008). Kübler-Ross identified five stages of grief that are commonly seen in persons who experience loss (Kübler-Ross, 1969). Losses ranging from the death of a loved one to the loss of a job can trigger the grief process. The five stages of Kübler-Ross's grief cycle include (1) denial, (2) anger, (3) bargaining, (4) depression, and (5) acceptance. Kübler-Ross described grief as an individual process, while Hamilton (2005) noted the fluidity and nonlinear nature of the grieving process (Hamilton, 2005; Kübler-Ross & Kessler, 2005). According to Kübler-Ross, people go through all, some, or none of the stages of grief and do so at their own pace. People may become stuck in a stage or recycle through a stage more than once. Kübler-Ross recognized that each person is different, that grief is an extremely personal experience, and that there is no certainty with regard to emotions or responses in each individual.

Healthcare patients are vulnerable to the stages of grief or loss because many experience loss of control, loss of their (personally defined) health, loss of quality of life, loss of independence, and possibly even loss of self-identity (Penzo & Harvey, 2008; Smart, 2008). Knowing if the patient is grieving and where the patient is in the grieving process can help the patient educator plan and execute patient teaching. Creating a supportive, respectful environment where patients feel heard and understood is important for their successful transition through grief. Understanding that grief is normal and may surface with any crisis throughout the patient's health management can help the patient educator be sensitive to each encounter with the patient (Hamilton, 2005; Penzo & Harvey, 2008).

EVOLUTION OF PATIENT INFORMATION

In the evolution of patient information, the patient moves from exposure through instruction to a level of individualization where ownership and control of information occurs. Exposure, the first function in the process of educating a patient, is the most common form of information-delivery seen in healthcare today and, unfortunately, is often mistaken for education. In exposure, information is given to the patient, but the preparation, delivery, and timing of information are all based on the provider's convenience and preference. Often, information is literally handed to the patient in a superficial and disconnected manner.

After the exposure level, a more concentrated level of instruction or teaching evolves, moving the communication process toward education and a more patient–centered process. From instruction, information progresses to patient ownership, where the patient processes information to include self. The addition of self to the information begins to individualize the information. Clarification and reinforcement, which can be achieved alone or in conjunction with the provider or educator, can help the patient prioritize new information and determine the influence that the new information will have on personal choices and behavior. After personal ownership of the information occurs, the patient can use the information to manipulate his personal world through choices based on information he personally possesses. Figure 7-3 displays the evolution of information in patient education.

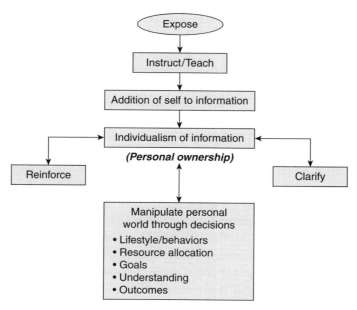

Figure 7-3. The progression of information in patient education. The process begins with exposure to teaching and instructing. From there, information can progress to where the recipient inserts self into the information. After the addition of self, information becomes individualized but maintains a need for occasional reinforcement or clarification. After individualism of information occurs, patients are empowered to manipulate their personal worlds through informed decision-making.

LEVELS OF KNOWLEDGE

The acquisition of knowledge is multifaceted. In academia, educators work hard to move students toward higher levels of knowing. Movement occurs in stages, grades, and at a variety of paces, resulting in students with varying levels of knowledge. As discussed in chapter 5, Bloom's taxonomy, a nomenclature of levels of human thought, is frequently used in academia. Bloom's taxonomy offers educators a guide to use as they determine where students need to be in regard to learning new information. The taxonomy assists educators in planning goals for a student's knowledge attainment and knowledge progression. Bloom's original taxonomy moved from the lowest level of thought—knowledge through comprehension, application, analysis, and synthesis—to evaluation, the highest level (Bloom, 1956). As students move from knowledge toward evaluation, their ability to comprehend and utilize information becomes more complex. Progressing up Bloom's taxonomy follows a student's mental transitioning of information from familiarity to ownership and, finally, to mastery.

In healthcare at present, mastery is rarely attained; exposure is where most patient-education attempts stop (Moons et al., 2001). This lack of focus on the progression of human thought has many implications; two are readily identified—safety and consent/informed decision. Patient education calls for a hierarchical approach to establish order in the patient's attainment of knowledge. Unlike with a traditional classroom student, lack of mastery in a patient can have life or death consequences (Osborne, 2005). The patient education hierarchy offers a focus for prioritizing a patient's knowledge needs (Figure 7-4). As the patient's knowledge migrates up the hierarchy, greater independence and self-determination are realized.

The hierarchy's foundational level focuses on safety. This level has to be achieved and maintained in order for any higher-level learning to occur. Maintaining safety will help to avoid preventable setbacks in health. Maintenance of safety allows the patient and healthcare provider to focus on health and knowledge progression. For example, teaching a patient how to ambulate safely and make sure pathways are well lit and uncluttered can help prevent falls and related injuries like fractures and sprains. Another example is safe medication administration, like alternating Coumadin dosages; making sure the patient understands how to administer Coumadin safely can help prevent too much or too little of the ordered dosage. Avoiding these potential safety hazards helps keep the patient's momentum moving toward improved health, maintains patient confidence,

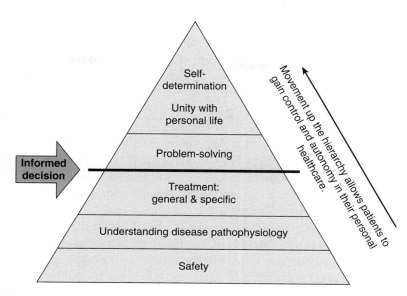

Figure 7-4. The patient education hierarchy provides a method with which to approach patient education prioritization. The foundational level of the hierarchy is safety. It is imperative that the patient always receives safety instruction first. From there, the patient progresses up the hierarchy to understanding the disease process, the treatment approach, and problem solving. The top level represents the ultimate goal of patient education—self-determination—where patient is in control of health inclusive of any disease state.

and allows the patient to concentrate on the next level of knowledge on the hierarchy.

The second level of the hierarchy, disease pathophysiology, offers the patient an opportunity to understand normal pathophysiology of the body and what is happening in his own body—chemically and physically—because of his health state. This understanding of physical and chemical circumstances helps to form a justification or rationale for the treatment plan. Understanding the "why" for the treatment plan helps ease the patient's knowledge-transition into the next level of the hierarchy. The third level entails the treatment that the patient is expected to follow. Treatment may include anything from a generic, universally-used treatment, such as daily weight-measurement for congestive heart failure patients, to a patient-specific treatment such as a prescribed heart-healthy diet regimen tailored to accommodate individual allergies.

Multiple reviews may be needed, but once patients understand the information, they have the knowledge base to actively participate in and regulate their care. Knowing the pathophysiology and treatment allows the patient to gain perspective into the healthcare provider's reasoning for formulating the treatment plan. A solid understanding of pathophysiology and treatment moves patients to a level where they should be comfortable making informed decisions regarding their care. Obtaining this level of knowledge can empower a patient with enough information to be able to ask questions, request clarification, acknowledge if the provider's conclusion is not congruent with their health state, reason-through treatment choices, and most importantly, personally advocate for self. This level of knowing moves a patient into an active role in the healthcare relationship by broadening his span of influence (see Chapter 4 for more detail).

Once the patient has made an informed decision, he will need to receive educational support to master the disease and treatment information. In mastering the disease and treatment information, problem solving should be applied to evaluate the patient's ability to react to and control predictable and unpredictable variables that could influence his health status. The fourth level—problem solving—requires in-depth understanding of the disease, complication management, and treatment protocol before the next level can be reached.

Once the skill of problem solving has been mastered, then the patient has reached the highest level of the hierarchy. In the highest level, the patient no longer sees the diagnosis as separate from self. The patient and the health state are one; the diagnosis has merged with the patient's identity. The patient controls the health state just as he does anything else in his life. Complete and full mastery of the health state allows understanding of the diagnosis to unify with sense of self. At the pinnacle of the hierarchy, the patient reaches a level of confidence and competence in self-care that transitions him to proficiency in knowing how to control and skillfully manage life choices and decisions. Through self-actualization, patients comfortably choose the progression and path for treatment that works best within their lives.

Today, patients with multiple chronic illnesses may be on various levels of the hierarchy at any given time. For example, a patient with diabetes, congestive heart failure, and recent stroke may be at the problem-solving level for diabetes, pathophysiology level for congestive heart failure, but only at the safety level for stroke. Dealing with acute situations versus chronic conditions may influence the patient's various levels of knowledge. The challenge for the healthcare provider is to balance the patients' knowledge progression while maintaining the foundational safety level. Safety should always be the first concern when approaching patient education. Lack of safety can negatively affect healthcare outcomes, levels of independence, and knowledge progression because of shifting focus from mental gain to physical gain.

Information should be structured so the patient progresses up the hierarchy toward the level where informed decision-making can be accomplished. This enables the patient to continue toward achieving full control of health status, as the knowledge becomes one with self. Once at the top level, self-determination begins as the patient has gained mastery of the health knowledge and unifies the health-state with self. The patient redefines self to include his new knowledge with all of his previous knowledge and skills. A new self emerges that is comprised of health conditions or diagnosis of illness as a part of self just like an arm or leg. No longer is the health state a burden or label. Instead, it is part of the person.

Information from the lower three levels of the hierarchy will always require reinforcement. Reinforcement helps to keep the information fresh and in the forefront of the patient's mind. The number of health conditions and diagnoses, along with personal health information season (discussed below), can impact a person's attainment of hierarchy-levels and knowledge progression.

INFORMATIONAL SEASONS OF KNOWLEDGE

Because of the magnitude of influence that information has in the provider-patient relationship, it is important to prepare patient information not only based on the receiver's understanding and retention needs, but also according to the direct personal impact of the health condition. In medagogy, three levels of health impact are used. These levels are referred to as *health informational seasons* (see Figure 7-5). Informational seasons offer a new way of looking at patient communication and learning. Seasons help the educator adjust the information to be delivered according to the position or place patients are at in their health.

Just as all patients are unique in their various needs, so is the timing of patient healthcare access.

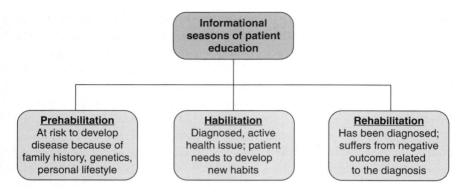

Figure 7-5. The three informational seasons of patient education. Prehabilitation is the season before disease onset or injury. Habilitation is the season where active diagnosis is made or a disease state (without the occurrence of deficits or injury) has occurred secondary to the diagnosis. Rehabilitation represents the season where negative insult has occurred because of the diagnosis or health state.

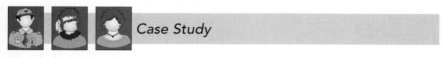

Case Study

Let's consider three patients: Michael, the local Boy Scout troop leader, is a patient with hypertension who now requires medication and a low-sodium diet. Marlene, the town's local artist and also a patient with hypertension, suffered a stroke secondary to her hypertension. Lastly, Phyllis, a young mother who works part-time as a cashier at the local market, has a family history of cardiovascular disease but no active diagnosis. All three individuals are at very different stages of health. All three patients are also at very different informational seasons in their health, even though they share the same actual or potential diagnosis: hypertension.

Given the variations in individual health seasons, it is important to capture each patient's season or timing by presenting information according to present health position on the continuum of the disease. Whether the patient is in the final days of living with a terminal illness, or if he runs the risk of developing a diagnosis because of personal or family history, the patient information needs to address the individual health season.

Medagogy identifies three informational seasons of patient education: (1) prehabilitation, (2) habilitation, and (3) rehabilitation. Each season offers a perspective for patient-education construction and delivery that helps make information more patient-centered and appropriate to the particular stage of personal health. Though the same information may be threaded throughout all seasons, the patient's unique position in correlation with the disease and is need to act helps to frame the information for that individual patient in his present situation. Each stage is named according to the patient's relationship to necessary health behavior changes. The seasons are independent of each other. Transition through one season is not contingent for progression into the next season. A person may transition through one or all of the seasons. It is the provider's responsibility to recognize a patient's health status relative to a season and to be capable of delivering information that is oriented appropriately.

 Case Study

Let's consider Michael, Marlene, and Phyllis again. All three patients share the same primary care physician, and they all coincidently accessed that provider on the same day. The information provided to each of them should be prepared based on where each individual is at in regard to their health. Although the same diagnosis, hypertension, is the focus of the education, each individual's health position should help the provider frame the focus of the patient-provider communication.

SEASON 1: PREHABILITATION

Prehabilitation is the season for prevention and promotion through patient education. During this phase, the patient is at risk for, or will develop, a diagnosis or health condition. The patient may have a strong family history, or his lifestyle may put him in jeopardy for developing or contracting a specific illness or health condition. In the preceding case study, Phyllis is in the prehabilitative season for hypertension because of her family history.

In the "at-risk-for" or prevention season, the healthcare provider appeals to the patient to change his behavior to reduce the odds of onset or risk of exposure. A smoking cessation course is an example of prehabilitation instruction to change behavior as a prevention technique. Prehabilitation instruction could also focus on gaining comfort and mastery of a skill or set of skills in preparation for the health state. Instruction about contraceptive measures for a non–sexually active person is an example of health promotion during prehabilitation. A Lamaze class for pregnant women is another an example of prehabilitation because it involves attaining a skill to be used for a future health state.

Patients' reactions to prehabilitation education are precarious because the pending health state or diagnosis is not yet a reality. The patient's only life experience with the disease or health condition may be through extension, exposure experienced through social networks, and observation of others. The person may have no experience with the health status and know nothing about the illness or condition. A pregnant woman who knows no one who has breastfed and knows nothing about breastfeeding is one example; she is in need of information that she may use after she delivers. The timing of her delivery may influence her motivation. The closer she is to her due date, the more motivated she may be to learn. Distance between the pending health status and the patient may offer a false sense of optimal health to the patient, leaving her with a lack of interest in the information that is being presented. Lack of urgency may reveal itself as procrastination or denial.

For the healthcare provider, patient engagement and commitment to action are the greatest challenges in the prehabilitation season. Any source of association, risk factors, or reality submersion should be utilized in relaying the relevance of the information and the need to act. For example, the type of breast cancer a patient's mother had puts her at risk for developing the same breast cancer. A strong family history of heart disease along with obesity and sedentary lifestyle puts a patient at higher risk for developing heart disease.

Communicating urgency in the information may spur motivation to learn and act. The link, the why-they-are-at-risk, must be present to support the prescribed behavior changes in order to delay or reduce risk of developing the pending health condition. The "why" offers a solid foundation on which to build a plan of action to address behavior and lifestyle.

A patient remains in the prehabilitation season of learning until a change in health status warrants the patient's movement into an active diagnosis or health insult state.

SEASON 2: HABILITATION

In the second season, habilitation, the patient has been diagnosed with the disease or health condition. The patient has an active diagnosis or insult to health and may or may not have associated symptoms. In the earlier case study, Michael is in the habilitative season for hypertension because his active diagnosis and treatment plan require an immediate change in diet and medication.

Just like patients in the prehabilitation season, patients in habilitation need to understand the "why" of the insult to their health status. The active status of the diagnosis in the habilitation season makes the goal of patient education focus on management of treatment for patient health. A solid understanding of the "why" will allow patients to master the management of their health state so they can avoid negative outcomes, exacerbation of symptoms, and further damage due to their health condition.

Patients may not have had any prior instruction related to their health condition, and this may be their first exposure to information regarding the diagnosis. If patient has prior knowledge about the disease, the next step is for the patient educator to find out what is known. It is important to note that *prior* knowledge does not mean *correct* knowledge. Clarification of misunderstood information is therefore very important and should be a top priority for the patient educator. If patient education begins without complete clarity of what is known and the assurance that the present understanding is correct, then patient education attempts may lead to chaos and confusion. The patient must possess accurate knowledge to build a solid and lasting understanding.

In the habilitation phase, patients may feel ambivalent about their diagnosis. Lack of any prior history, either personal or familial, along with vagueness or absence of symptoms may serve to heighten any reservations the patient may have about the diagnosis. The healthcare provider's diagnosis or confirmation of change in the patient's health status may act as a catalyst, triggering patient entry into a grieving process. Grief and loss may occur because of patients' perceptions about their loss of desired health and well-being (Penzo & Harvey, 2008). The patient may grieve the loss of health and/or the perceived loss of self. Even the temporary need for healthcare treatment or lifestyle changes may trigger a sense of loss of control and quality of life, initiating the possibility of the patient moving through some, all, or perhaps none of the grief cycle. Each stage of grief the patient moves through offers a new challenge to information-delivery in the habilitation season.

The key to success in the habilitation season is to support the patient as he moves through emotions associated with an alteration in health, and to be prepared when the patient is emotionally ready to move toward a plan. The goal is for the patient's information to be delivered by the healthcare team at a level the patient understands so that the patient is able to utilize the information. Through work, patience, and acceptance, the patient may be able to move beyond understanding to control and merge information into his life.

Ultimately, the provider should strive to help patients reach a level where self-determination is influenced by personal disease understanding, allowing the diagnosis to become a part of self and no longer viewed as something extra or different. The secret to reaching self-determination lies in the healthcare provider-patient relationship and the independence of the patient. Just as the healthcare provider assumes the role of expert of health, likewise the patient should be viewed as the expert of self. The disease understanding that is shared between the two experts is shared knowledge on which the patient's treatment is planned by the two experts. This shared knowledge will also serve as a foundation for all future disease information.

Shared knowledge unites the disease information provided by the healthcare provider like (disease pathophysiology and treatment) with a patient's individual information (values and lifestyle). The shared knowledge serves as a foundation for a true partnership between healthcare provider and patient. With shared knowledge, both parties must accept and understand each other's perspective and expertise, while at the same time offering personal perspectives and desires. Shared knowledge empowers both patient and provider with a voice to offer and discuss opinions, suggestions, and address any issues that could affect treatment compliance.

As commonly used, the term *compliance* is generic and misleading, while its counterpart *noncompliance* bears a pejorative tone (Shea, 2006). Compliance no longer means trying to force the patient into a pre-established optimal disease treatment box. Instead, discussion and planning between the patient and the provider helps formulate a mutual treatment consensus. Compliance no longer represents conformity to one perspective, but instead becomes the fulfillment of each individual's responsibility to an agreed-upon treatment strategy. Movement from the planned course is no longer seen as noncompliance or capricious misconduct, but instead is seen as an action based on an informed decision (Shea, 2006). Such intelligent noncompliance then flags the experts to review and rethink the treatment plan (Trostle, 1988). Noncompliance is replaced with choice and informed decision-making.

Patients remain in the habilitation season of learning until their diagnosis or health state is no longer active or resolves, or until negative health outcomes occur. If negative effects occur or health declines to the extent that adaptations are needed for regular activities of daily living, then the patient moves into the rehabilitative informational season. An example of this is a hypertensive patient who has a stroke with complete left-sided residual deficit. The patient might require training on ambulation, feeding, and basic activities of living; this training is the focus of the rehabilitation season.

SEASON 3: REHABILITATION

Patient teaching that occurs in the rehabilitation season focuses on empowering patients with knowledge that can help them accommodate functional deficits that have occurred secondary to the development and progression of a disease state. In the earlier case study (page 113), Marlene is in the rehabilitation season. Marlene is learning to accommodate for the physical deficits she acquired related to her stroke.

Grief is an issue the patient educator can expect to encounter in the rehabilitation season just as in the habilitation season. In the rehabilitative season, grieving is focused on the loss of perceived individual normalcy or self-image, changes in the routine of personal life, and fear of death and dying. If the health insult is severe enough, then loss of independence may also be a major issue for not only the patient, but for caregivers and family as well.

This phase can occur during a time of major life crisis as the patient tries to sort through options. It is important that information be direct, factual, and reinforced. If the patient has had an opportunity to progress through prior seasons, prehabilitation and habilitation, this may help provide a foundation on which to build new information. If the patient has not had prehabilitation and/or habilitation instruction, then building a solid foundation about what is occurring in the body and correlating symptoms or outcomes with pathophysiology is required to provide the "why" for the patient to understand risks, options, and prospective treatment.

If an insult to the brain has occurred, such as a stroke, the patient may not be able to recall any previous instruction received. The goal then concentrates on redeveloping a solid foundation of knowledge upon which effective treatment plans can be constructed. Family is likely to be present and at the patient's side because of negative effects from the condition that have placed the patient in the rehabilitative season. In the rehabilitative season, the focus of education is on learning to live with and accommodate for deficits resulting from health-status insult. The insult may be temporary, but until full recovery is attained, the focus is on making sure that no further injury occurs because of disease or diagnosis.

Family members can be helpful and can serve as advocates for the patient. The focus of all instruction should remain patient-centered, making certain that the patient understands. Caregivers, spouses, or those who will be responsible for patients while they are incapacitated and dependent on someone else must be taught just as if they were patients. These individuals will also need to understand clearly that although they are not patients, they must strive to help providers meet the patients' preferences and needs. Success in following through with treatment relies on patients and caregivers understanding the treatment specifics. Ultimately, the goal is to make the patient as independent as possible by helping the patient and caregivers understand how to manage the disease/health status and the self-care that will be needed for quality of life.

Rehabilitation may become so manageable that the patient may move back to the habilitation season where the focus of education is on management and prevention of negative outcomes. Prehabilitation can also be re-entered if there is a risk for another health status change or disease because of the primary condition that triggered the negative symptoms or outcomes. Patients may cross over all three of the information seasons depending on their health status or in the case of multiple diagnoses. The most important thing is for the patient educator to know what informational season the patient is in so that information can be adjusted to accommodate the patient, instead of the patient accommodating the information. Just as public health utilizes primary, secondary and tertiary to define levels of care, medagogy employs the informational seasons to classify patient knowledge needs in relation to immediacy of health alteration. Informational seasons of patient education are an integral part of the medagogy framework.

Case Study

Janet is a 36-year-old Native American female who works as a librarian at the town library. She has a history of morbid obesity and hypertension, and recently elected to undergo bariatric surgery. She has been prepared for her new diet and lifestyle through multiple preoperative visits. Now that Janet has had the surgery, she is in pain and is suffering from extreme bouts of nausea and vomiting. The food she had purchased preoperatively to eat when she returned home from surgery is not settling well with her "new" stomach. Because Janet understands the risk of malnutrition with bariatric surgery, she decides she needs to call her surgeon for direction. Although Janet worries about "bothering" her surgeon, she feels that since her present state is not improving she must do something. Janet's high insurance co-pay for emergency room visits also serves as an impetus for the physician call.

After calling the surgeon, Janet felt comfortable that she knew what to do to help decrease her nausea and vomiting. Janet's appropriate actions of accessing the healthcare system through her surgeon (primary care for this issue) saved her from suffering potential negative consequences like dehydration or electrolyte imbalance. Janet's functional understanding of the surgery she underwent, as well as her astuteness in correlating the prospective consequence her emesis could ultimately have on her health, empowered Janet to act independently and appropriately. Without Janet's early intervention she may have been hospitalized, costing her more time and money to address an issue that was preventable.

MOVING FORWARD

In the 1500s, toward the later years of his life, the Italian architect Michelangelo Buonarroti stated "Ancora impero" as he referenced his accomplished works. In 1847, Ralph Waldo Emerson, in his book *Poetry and Imagination,* translated the famous architect's words as "I am still learning." The phrase "Ancora impero" has been interpreted as "I continue to learn" (Bucy, 1981) and "still I am learning" (Emerson, 1912). Regardless of the specific translation, the sentiment of being subject to perpetual learning is of relevance to both patients and patient educators. Individual health is an art of study that requires all parties to assume the role of life-long learner.

The new era of value-based healthcare purchasing and Hospital Consumer Assessment of Healthcare Providers Systems (HCAHPS) measures will demand a knowledgeable patient. As healthcare moves forward, patient education must be included as an essential component of healthcare delivery. Transitioning providers and patients to assume a teaching and learning focus with every healthcare interaction presents the need for direction. Evolution of patient information, patient education hierarchy, and informational seasons of patient education are concepts that help construct the framework of medagogy. Medagogy serves to provide direction for the artful skill of patient education.

SUMMARY

- Aristotle, in his first book of *Metaphysics*, asserted that the main difference between master craftsmen and manual workers lies in the former's grasp of the theory underlying their work. Aristotle posits that within the understanding of "why" lies reason, which provides an insight or wisdom that can be used beyond the immediate intended utility.

- The art and science of educating patients has traditionally consisted of the provider finding the fit, mode, and method of information delivery that worked best for the individual provider.

- Experts argue that unskilled communication by healthcare providers is to blame for their poor performance in patient education. Schwartzenburg and colleagues assert that healthcare professionals need to be trained in how to teach.

- The uniqueness of the patient as a student creates the need to look at patient education as a special form of education, separate from traditionally held mainstream ideas about education that primarily occurs in academic institutions.

- The licensed healthcare provider serves as a subject matter expert (e.g., health, healthcare, treatment, and disease). The patient, on the other hand, serves as an expert of self in the patient-provider relationship.

- Information needs to be openly exchanged in the provider-patient relationship. Information withheld from either party could directly impact potential outcomes.

- In healthcare at present, mastery is rarely attained because exposure is where most patient education attempts stop.

- Knowing the pathophysiology and treatment allows the patient to gain perspective into the reasoning used by the healthcare provider to formulate the treatment plan. A solid understanding of pathophysiology and treatment moves the patient to a level where they should be comfortable making informed decisions regarding their care.

- Higher levels of knowing moves patients into a more active role in the healthcare relationship by broadening their span of influence.

- In self-actualization, patients are able to comfortably choose the progression and path for treatment within their life.

- In medagogy, three levels of health impact are used. These levels are referred to as health informational seasons. Informational seasons offer a new way of looking at patient communication and learning. Seasons help the educator adjust information to be delivered according to the position patients are at regarding their health.

- Medagogy identifies three informational seasons of patient education: (1) prehabilitation, (2) habilitation, and (3) rehabilitation.

- Each season is named according to the patient's relationship to necessary health behavior changes. The seasons are independent of each other.

- Prehabilitation is the season for prevention and health-promotion through patient education. During this phase, the patient is at risk for, or will develop, a diagnosis or health condition.

- Patients' reactions to prehabilitation education are precarious because the pending health state or diagnosis is not yet a reality.

- In habilitation, the patient has been diagnosed with a disease or health condition. The patient has an active diagnosis or insult to health and may or may not have associated symptoms. The active status of the diagnosis makes the goal of the season to educate patients in the management or treatment of their health-condition.

- The key to success in the habilitation season is to support patients as they move through emotions associated with an alteration in health, and to be prepared when the patient is emotionally ready to move toward a plan.

- Patients remain in the habilitation season of learning until their diagnosis or health state is no longer active, resolves, or until negative health outcomes occur.

- Patient teaching that occurs in the rehabilitation season focuses on empowering patients with knowledge that can help them accommodate functional deficits that have occurred secondary to the development and progression of a disease state. This phase can occur during a time of major life crisis as the patient tries to sort through options. It is important that information be direct, factual, and reinforced.

- It is normal for patients to experience a wide array of emotions while receiving healthcare. Emotions add a significant challenge to patient learning. The emotion factor is a unique characteristic common to the patient-pupil.

- Understanding that grief is normal and may surface with any crisis throughout the patient's healthcare-management process can help the patient educator be sensitive during each encounter with the patient.

[CHAPTER 8]

The Brain and Memory

This chapter will shift focus to human memory and the work of the brain in making memories. First, concepts of memory will be covered then emotional links will be reviewed. How educators can capitalize on the brain's capabilities will be discussed follow by the effects of information flow.

MEMORY

Recall that in Chapter 5 one of the oldest laws of learning was reviewed: the law of exercise (Thorndike, 1932). The law of exercise is based on the concept that repetition of information progresses that information through the stages of memory. The more a person hears the same information, the greater the chance he has of mentally filing that information away to be retrieved when needed (Feldman & McPhee, 2008; Ormrod, 2008). A review of how memory works may help patient educators better understand how to maximize a person's memory potential.

To create a memory, three processes must occur (Klein, 2009). First, the occurrence must deposit as a memory. Next, the memory must be of value to morph with previously stored memories. Lastly, the brain must evoke the memory (Klein, 2009). Human memory is divided into three different stages: immediate, short-term, and long-term. Immediate memory has a duration of two seconds or less (Higbee, 2001; Minninger, 1997; Sousa, 2006). Immediate memory occurs when external input is initially stored through sensory impression (Feldman & McPhee, 2008). A variety of generalities may be involved in the memory, such as the color of one's eyes, name, clothing or outfit, laugh, spouse, location of meeting, and who was standing beside the person (Higbee, 2001). As the moment of registering passes, details of the impression start to fade, leaving only significant remnants of data (Higbee, 2001; Feldman & McPhee, 2008). Immediate memory is also referenced as sensory memory or working memory. If information that enters into the immediate memory does not have value or meaning to the receiver, then the information is discarded and forgotten. However, if the data does bear significance, then it will progress to the next level of memory—the short-term memory.

Short-term memory has a duration lasting from 30 seconds to two days (Higbee, 2001; Minniger, 1997). The universally accepted limit of the capacity for short-term memory is seven items (Cowan, 2001; Feldman & McPhee, 2008; Klein, 2009; MacGregor, 1987). The first study to identify a capacity for short-term memory was Miller's 1956 study, where findings suggested that seven chunks, plus or minus two, constituted the approximate capacity of the short-term memory (Miller, 1956). Chunks are information grouped according to personal significance (Miller, 1956). The capacity of the short-term memory remains controversial. At present, an empirically supported range from four to seven is accepted (Chase & Simon, 1973; Cowan, 2001; Miller, 1956). Short-term memory links information for long-term storage together through context and the assignment of meaning to information (Higbee, 2001; Klein, 2009). Short-term memory is an active process. Only through the work of rehearsal or repetition can information be transitioned from short-term memory to long-term memory (Feldman & McPhee, 2008; Klein, 2009).

Long-term memory has infinite capacity and limitless duration (Feldman & McPhee, 2008; Klein, 2009; Sousa, 2006). Once information is stored in the long-term memory, it is divided into two areas: declarative and nondeclarative. Declarative or explicit information is further subdivided as episodic or semantic memory. Episodic memory includes memories of events, life history, and personal lived moments in time (Feldman & McPhee, 2008). Episodic memories form, store, and recall with ease. Positive feelings associated with a memory can help strengthen it (Feldman & McPhee, 2008). Semantic or declarative memory is the conglomeration of facts and data not related to any event. Declarative memory is the memory most associated with school and learning. These memories are "easy-come, easy-go" memories. The use of rehearsal, repetition, or mnemonics is required to strengthen declarative memory (Feldman & McPhee, 2008).

Nondeclarative memory, or implicit memory, is procedural information. Nondeclarative memory is the "how-to" memory that is used in the attainment of procedural skill sets (Feldman & McPhee, 2008, p.93). Nondeclarative memory is used in the preparation of all licensed health-care providers and is used every day in the execution of professional tasks and responsibilities. Nondeclarative memories include skills like irrigating a suction tube, starting an intravenous line, and conducting an interview. Nondeclarative memories are hard to form and are learned through conditioning and reinforcement, but will last for years (Bauer, 1996; Feldman & McPhee, 2008). Practice can make memories. Retention of information can occur through rote rehearsal, practice, and repetition (Higbee, 2001). A specific sequence of information repeatedly revisited can help make connections with already present or stored information (Feldman & McPhee, 2008, MacGregor, 1987, Minninger, 1997). The repeated information reinforces meaning, while present connections guide new information in learning and, of course, memory.

EMOTIONAL LINKS

Plato once said, "All learning has an emotional base" (Feldman and McPhee, 2008, p. 321). A learner brings beliefs, values, and interests to the learning experience, all of which have personal significance. Emotional centers of the brain are interwoven with the cognitive learning areas of the brain (Zins, Weissberg, Wang, & Walberg, 2004). Meaning is linked to emotion (Feldman and McPhee, 2008). Learning can be emotionally promoted in two ways: by establishing a personal emotional learning climate and by triggering memories from information taught. Personal emotional climate refers to the moods of learners while they are ingesting and processing information (Jensen, 2000). A positive emotional state, especially about learning, can aid in the learning process (Feldman & McPhee, 2008). A comfortable learning environment can help the learner relax, which can facilitate learning and enhance memory (Jensen, 2000; Sousa, 2006).

Memories evoked may stimulate emotions through the memory's connections. The term *flashbulb memories,* coined by Brown and Kulik in 1977, refers to vivid memories of circumstances under which someone first learns of shocking, momentous, emotionally charged information. The information is stored once but remembered for a lifetime (Jensen, 2000). Flashbulb memories are very reliable memories and are often associated with events like the Oklahoma bombing, the World Trade Center attack, and the deaths of leaders like Princess Diana, Martin Luther King, and

President Kennedy. The relationship between instructor and student can also stimulate emotions that can affect learning. Emotions can serve as reinforcement or a barrier, and understanding and mastering their use can help the educator in relaying information that can be remembered. As mentioned previously, positive memories can enhance learning and negative memories can seal memories through the emotional charge (Jensen, 2000; Klein, 2009). The likelihood and the accuracy of memories stored in a negatively charged emotional climate are influenced by the personal relationship to the information or news (Klein, 2009).

Learning alters the brain. The brain physically changes for memory storage. Permanent memories are formed when the same stimulus repeatedly causes a network of neurons to fire together (Klein, 2009; Zull, 2006). Increased neuron-signaling generates growth of more neural branches, increases the density of the area, and stimulates more synapses (Zull, 2006). Repeated firing of a neural network eventually results in the ability to stimulate one neuron in the network, which causes the firing of the entire network, which in turn triggers the recall of the associated memory (Zull, 2006). This process helps to prevent cluttering of useless information in the long-term memory. When memories are made, the neural forest actually moves, morphing as new information joins with already present information (Zull, 2006).

The goal of patient educators should be to move information regarding diagnosis or health status from immediate memory through short-term memory into the patient's long-term memory. An understanding of the stages of memory in the brain as well as how to assist the patient in the reception, processing, and storing of information in the learning process should be a part of an educator's repertoire of knowledge. Knowing how the brain makes memories can help the patient educator to establish an environment conducive to learning. The role of patient, disease, and/or insult can cause a deficit in the functioning of cognitive areas that can negatively affect patient learning. Knowledge of cognitive operational functioning during learning and memory construction can aid the patient educator in planning instruction while taking into consideration cognitive limitations resulting from disease or insult.

Long-term memory serves as a reservoir for personal knowledge. Speed and accuracy of memory retrieval is contingent on both encoding and the attributes of the memory (Ormrod, 2008). Memory attributes may ascribe affective (emotional) or contextual (circumstantial) phenomena encountered during the memory event (Albon, 2008; Ormrod, 2008). Retrieval of stored memories occurs through free or cued recall (Albon,

2008; Eddy, 2007; Zins, Weissberg, Wang, & Walberg, 2004). Free recall in memory transpires without cues (Eddy, 2007), whereas cued recall occurs in response to reminders of the memory (Albon, 2008, Ormrod, 2008).

Once information has been encoded into long-term memory, the objective is for a person to recall the stored information for personal use. Unfortunately, decay, a process where psychologists assume that memories fade, may conflict with the notion of the long-term memory's capacity to hold lifetime memories. Psychologists believe that most of the intricate details of memories fade in the decaying process (Ormrod, 2008). Ormrod (2008) asserts that some memories may simply be misfiled, whereas unused memories may get lost and become less accessible. Educators can assist in memory retrieval by providing clues and hints or details surrounding the memory event (Ormrod, 2008; Sousa, 2006). Retrieving memories is important for patient educators so they can know what a patient knows. New knowledge-construction needs to be built on a reliable foundation of understanding (Redman, 2001).

CAPITALIZING ON BRAIN CAPABILITIES

Education designed to capitalize on brain processes and capabilities is referred to as "teaching to the brain." These techniques focus on methods that will help the learner in receiving, processing, filing, and recalling information. Teaching with brain processing and cognitive storage in mind makes sense, especially in healthcare where time is limited and understanding and application treatment is critical. Unlike in grade school, healthcare providers do not have one hour a day, 180 days a year, to progress patients toward understanding their health. Therefore, every interaction with the patient has to include health information that the patient will be able to understand, retain, and use. Framing teaching efforts to maximize the brain's ability to understand and process information for storage and personal retrieval helps to alleviate possible errors in information-coding and transfer (Higbee, 2001; Jensen, 2000).

One technique of teaching to the brain is based on the fact that people learn information they have previously been exposed to faster than information they have never before been exposed to (Feldman & McPhee, 2008; Jensen, 2000; Klein, 2009; Ormrod, 2008). Before initiating patient teaching, first ask patients what they know about the information or topic about to be discussed. Listen for two things in their response: (1) Does the patient have a foundational understanding of what they need to know?

That is, does there exist a solid understanding to which new information can be added? (2) Does the patient understand what is is physically or chemically happening in his body relative to the disease?

 Case Study

Haddie is a retired cafeteria worker who is 67 years old, widowed, lives alone, and has been diagnosed with congestive heart failure (CHF) for 10 years. On evaluation of Haddie's present understanding of her health status, specifically CHF, she verbalizes as she places her hand to her chest that her "congestive heart failure" (which she says correctly) involves her heart. Haddie goes on to say that to help her heart she takes a fluid pill every evening that makes her get up two to three times a night to go to the bathroom. When asked "Anything else?" Haddie says, "Nope, that's all, if I take my pill I can breathe. If not, then I can't." Figure 8-1 represents Haddie's thought processes while she was talking about her fluid pill.

In the preceding case study, Haddie is able to correlate the relationship between the medication and the control of disease symptomology—breathlessness—as well as the relationship between the pill and frequent use of the bathroom at night. Overall, Haddie shares minimal knowledge for someone who has lived with CHF for 10 years, but what Haddie relates does provide some insight into her personal understanding of the disease and her treatment. The information offered is correct. Figure 8-2 represents the healthcare provider's thought processes while Haddie was telling her about her fluid pill.

It is important to determine if the information is erroneous in any way. For example, Haddie might have misunderstood CHF to mean any of the following:

- Diagnosis involving her bladder—that is why she urinates frequently at night.
- Normal with seasonal changes—cold medications always list congestion.

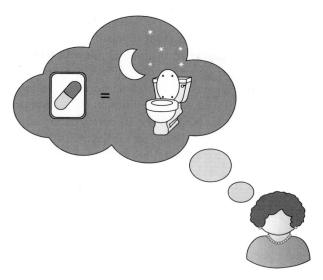

Figure 8-1.   The illustration displays Haddie's thought related to her fluid pill and what happens when she takes her pill.

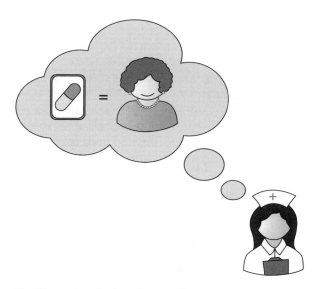

Figure 8-2.   The illustration displays the nurse's thought of Haddie's fluid-pill regimen and its relationship to a happy, healthy Haddie.

Alternatively, Haddie might have misunderstood her medication (fluid pill) information as indicated by the following:

- Her pill is only needed when she is breathless.
- Her pill will heal her heart.

Any misunderstanding of health status or treatment must be addressed before more information is added. The patient educator needs to connect the patient's perception to correct understanding so the patient, the educator, and the team of healthcare providers share complementary understanding of the patient's health. Time and effort must be invested in using the information that is known, clarifying any misperceptions, and making certain that the resulting understanding is correct and usable. Any additional knowledge-building must be suspended until corrections and clarifications are made and understood. This may appear to be a step backward to some providers, but this period of clarification and correcting should instead be viewed as partnering with the patient through investing personal knowledge and insight in the patient's health. Figure 8-3 represents the initial thoughts of the patient and the educator or provider when the term *heart* is spoken. The

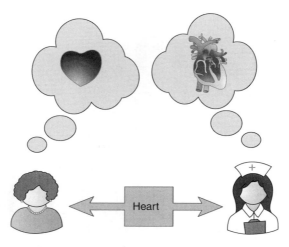

Figure 8-3. The figure displays the separate thoughts of the patient and the nurse when each thinks of the heart. The patient thinks of a pretty Valentine heart, while the provider visualizes an anatomically correct heart and its functionality.

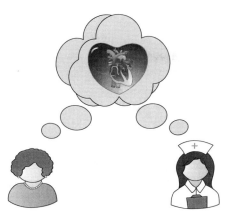

Figure 8-4. The figure shows the merging of the two independent perspectives to create shared knowledge. With shared knowledge the patient has an understanding of the provider's knowledge of the heart, and the provider has an understanding of the patient's knowledge of the heart.

figure displays the patient's thought as an average layperson image of a heart, like a Valentine heart, whereas the patient educator thinks of an anatomically correct working heart. In Figure 8-4, the thoughts merge because of shared knowledge between the provider/patient educator and the patient.

 ## Case Study

In another example of reconstructing prior knowledge, Julie, a 21-year-old single female who is six months pregnant with her first child, has chosen not to attend any of the free prenatal and Lamaze classes offered. Julie states that she is familiar with labor and the pain of contractions even though this is her first pregnancy. Julie states that she knows that a breathing technique can completely alleviate the pain because her sister Joyce has had three children naturally with no drugs. Julie asserts that if it worked for Joyce, then it will work for her.

Many challenges are present for the patient educator in Julie's scenario. First, correcting the misunderstanding that pain is removed through a breathing technique needs to be addressed. While the labor pain may be controlled somewhat, complete alleviation through breathing alone is unrealistic. When addressing the patient's understanding of contractions, the patient educator should respect Julie's value of her sister's experience while preparing Julie for the physical changes that occur in the body during a contraction and how people have stated the contraction felt. Exposing the patient to what physically occurs in a laboring woman's body will help to provide a factual understanding of what is actually happening during a contraction cycle. Understanding what is occurring in the body allows the patient access to information used by the health expert—the healthcare provider (Boren, Wakefield, Gunlock, & Wafefield, 2009). Learning information about the body's physical and chemical processes enables the patient to gain insight into the knowledge that drives healthcare providers' decisions (Williams, Lindsell, Rue, & Blomkalns, 2007). Understanding "why" helps establish a foundational rationale, which can be an asset in treatment decisions for the provider and the patient (Tokarz, 2009). When patients need to make decisions regarding treatment options that have been offered, if they have been exposed to rationale they should be able to support choices made.

Simply smiling and handing over a pamphlet cannot prepare patients for an active role in their healthcare treatment in the same way as one-on-one instruction about the body's physical and chemical functions. This instruction helps to heighten patients' awareness as to where they are on the health continuum (Hernandez, Balter, Bourbeau, & Hodder, 2009). A provider's expertise in healthcare can serve as a resource for issues patients may have questions about. Resource-access to meet the patient's informational needs should be made available to the patient. Once patients make informed decisions and are secure in their choices, they should be supported free of judgment or criticism. Debating personal or professional position is not of any value after a decision has been made, and should be discouraged.

When educating patients, avoid negative terminology and remarks such as "cannot" or "does not." This will help the brain in the mental processing of the information (Calvin, 1995; Given, 2002; Sousa, 2006). When negative statements like "cannot" or "does not" are processed mentally, the information has to be reverted to the positive, can or does, before the negative can be added (Calvin, 1995). After the information is transitioned twice, then it can be stored (Calvin, 1995). With negative terminology, the process includes receiving the negative information, reversing the information to positive, reversing information back to the negative information again, and finally, storing the information. The extra steps involved in processing negative statements increase the odds of mis-filing the information, which heightens the odds of misunderstanding the information.

Negatives can be taught by first creating the positive flow of thought, then adding the negative thought after the positive is filed. By first initiating positive thoughts like "can" and "does," then adding the nega-tive of "not," the brain only has to add the negative without having to switch the information independently. Another approach to avoiding negatives is to avert the use of terminology such as, "to avoid this" or "to prevent that from happening." Alternatively, allowing the relationship of negative to be imposed by self-discovery, such as with dieting education, is another option. Examples such as "calorie intake is important," "for weight loss a 1200-calorie diet is recommended," "anything over 1200 calories will be stored as fat," and "fat stored will increase weight," pro-vide understanding so the negatives can be assumed or discovered by the receiver.

When evaluating a patient's presenting knowledge, it is important to assess the patient's understanding of what is physically or chemically happening in his body (Boren, Wakefield, Gunlock, & Wafefield, 2009; Redman, 2007; Williams, Lindsell, Rue, & Blomkalns, 2007). Expectation of a textbook understanding is not realistic, but a rough depiction of what is happening can serve the educator well in efforts to progress the patient's knowledge (Redman, 2007). In keeping with the building con-struction analogy, any solid construction has a logical order or sequence (Greenburg, 1991; Ormrod, 2008; Redman, 2007; Sousa, 2006). Builders know when they need to hang the front door for a house. The front door is not hung before the foundation, before the walls, and especially before the doorframe. For solid quality construction there is a time for every stage of construction and for every part of the house. The same is true with patient education. There is a time and a stage for every piece of information if we want to build a solid understanding that can serve throughout a lifetime of health. A solid foundational understanding will allow a lifetime of knowledge construction to occur. Additions and reno-vations maybe needed, but the builder knows the plans and a solid struc-ture will be able to handle it.

SUMMARY

- The law of exercise is based on the concept that repetition of information progresses that information through the stages of memory. The more often a person is exposed to the same information, the greater the chance he has of mentally filing that information in a way that can be retrieved when needed. A review of how memory works may help patient educators to better understand how they can maximize a person's memory potential.

- Short-term memory has a duration lasting from 30 seconds to two days.

- Short-term memory links information for long-term storage together through context and the assignment of meaning to information. Short-term memory is an active process. Only through the work of rehearsal or repetition can information be transitioned from short-term memory to long-term memory.

- Practice can make memories. Retention of information can occur through rote rehearsal, practice, and repetition. A specific sequence of information repeatedly revisited can help make connections with already present or stored information.

- Repeated information reinforces meaning, while present connections guide new information in learning and, of course, memory.

- Memories evoked may stimulate emotions through the memory's connections.

- Positive memories can enhance learning, and negative memories can seal memories through the emotional charge. The likelihood and the accuracy of memories stored in a negatively charged emotional climate are influenced by the personal relationship to the information or news.

- The goal of patient educators should be to move information regarding diagnosis or health status from immediate memory through short-term memory into the patient's long-term memory. Knowing how the brain makes memories can help the patient educator to establish an environment conducive to learning.

- Once information has been encoded into long-term memory, the objective is for a person to recall the stored information for personal use.

- Education designed to capitalize on brain processes and capabilities is referred to as "teaching to the brain." These techniques focus on methods that will help the learner in receiving, processing, filing, and recalling information.

- One technique of teaching to the brain is based on the fact that people learn information they have previously been exposed to faster than information they have never before been exposed to.

- Any misunderstanding of health status or treatment must be addressed before more information is added. The patient educator needs to connect the patient's perception to correct understanding so the patient, the educator, and the team of healthcare providers share complementary understanding of the patient's health.

- Simply smiling and handing over a pamphlet cannot prepare patients for an active role in their healthcare treatment in the same way as one-on-one instruction about the body's physical and chemical functions.

- A provider's expertise in healthcare can serve as a resource for the patient on information they may have questions about. Resources to meet patient's informational needs should be made available to the patient.

- There is a time and a stage for every piece of information if we want to have a solid understanding that can serve throughout a lifetime of health. A solid foundational understanding will allow a lifetime of knowledge construction to occur.

SECTION III SUMMARY

When is the last time you heard a layperson say, "Well I'm off to the hospital to learn"? When the general public reflects on healthcare, they often think of finding answers to issues they are dealing with while in an environment where people take care of them. Providers reference common patient educational efforts as instructions, whereas patients frequently reference providers teaching-efforts as being told what to do. When a layperson thinks of education and learning, academic schools are what come to mind—not healthcare. But evidence has shown that for optimal health outcomes to be achieved, patients need to learn while they are receiving and/or following healthcare treatment. Health prevention and maintenance cannot occur intentionally without a knowledgeable patient. The new era of value-based healthcare purchasing and Hospital Consumer Assessment of Healthcare Providers Systems (HCAHPS) measures demand a knowledgeable patient.

Providers of healthcare bring a wealth of knowledge related to the human body and actions that may impact health to the patient-provider relationship. It is important that providers are able to effectively assist patients in gaining understanding about their health status and treatment choices. Recognition that learning is an individualized process and that patients bring unique circumstances to the educational experience can help establish realistic information-exchange. As patients navigate the healthcare system, each provider and access-point offers new opportunities for learning. Skill in the teaching and learning process can aid providers as they communicate vital information to patients. As patients master information regarding their health, they can increase their health autonomy and progress to a point where self-determination can be attained. Knowledge of health status coupled with self-expertise empowers patients as they move toward optimal health.

Medagogy's health informational seasons serve to help educators orient health information in relation to patient proximity to health status and health consequences. The prehabilitation season is where a person is at risk for health implications, while in the habilitation season the patient has a diagnosis or an alteration in health status but has suffered no residual insult. The season of rehabilitation distinguishes a phase where the patient has endured an insult that has lingering consequences secondary to the altered health status. Patients' entry into and movement throughout the health informational seasons are not predictive or sequential.

No matter where patients are in their health, they deserve to have information from their health providers that they can understand, remember, and use. Patient teaching needs to be clear and purposeful. Patient educators can facilitate movement of information from immediate memory through short-term memory into long-term memory. Understanding how the brain learns can help facilitate learning as patients receive, process, file, and recall information. Insuring that information delivered is encoded correctly can help the receiver properly file data stored in the brain. Information can be accessed more easily when it is filed appropriately. To ensure a solid foundation of understanding, incorrect or misunderstood information should be corrected before new information is added. A solid foundation of understanding will allow for a lifetime of knowledge construction to occur. Making sure that information is effectively distributed can facilitate patient learning and comprehension as patients navigate along the healthcare continuum.

SECTION IV

INFORMATION DELIVERY METHODOLOGY

[CHAPTER 9]

The PITS Model

This section of the book will introduce the PITS model, the medagogy Conceptual Framework and conclude with the Understanding Personal Perspective Scale (UPP). The reader will move through the rationale and foundational philosophy supporting the PITS model into direct application of the model in practice. After reviewing PITS we will transition into an overview of the medagogy Conceptual Framework followed by an example of the framework's use in the CMS Care Transition's pilot. The section will conclude with the UPP scale, a new evaluation methodology that allows patients to quantify their knowledge and ability to act. The universal application of this tool offers hope in attacking the problem of health literacy.

Information needs to flow logically so it can be received, filed, and retrieved easily. When behavior modification is the goal, providing a "why" up front can ease the patient's confusion (Jensen, 2000; Redman, 2007). Not understanding the reason for change can make any alteration in behavior difficult to comply with or agree to (Jensen, 2009: Redman, 2007). Presenting information in an organized and logical format can enhance the receiver's ability to recall the information (Given, 2002; Slavin, 1995; Sousa, 2006), and also enables the receiver to easily follow the educator's train of thought (Slavin, 1995; Sousa, 2006). When information is composed of pieces and parts that are randomly distributed, the receiver is forced to assimilate and organize the information before it can be mentally filed. Leaving the task of organizing the information completely to the receiver creates room for error, misfiling, and misunderstanding (Given, 2002; Greenburg, 1991; Redman, 2007).

Organizing information into categories can enhance learning (Feldman & McPhee, 2008; Sousa, 2006). Adding logical order to information for patients does not have to be difficult. Redman (2007) points out that information needs to be delivered in an orderly, sequential style according to the patient's need. Stewart suggests that information should flow either from disease toward the patient or away from the patient toward disease. The direction of information-flow may be contingent on the emotional state of the patient or upon time constraints. For example, consent for emergency surgery may require information to flow from disease toward patient. In this situation, the surgeon starts with an explanation of what is happening in the body, what treatment options are available, what lifestyle implications may result, and that consent is needed if surgery is to happen immediately. In contrast, a person having an acute crisis, such as an asthma attack, may need information to flow from patient toward disease. That is, information-delivery would start with treatments the patient needs to know and do now and work back toward how the treatment will affect the internal functioning of the body and the disease.

PITS PATIENT EDUCATION INFORMATIONAL DELIVERY MODEL

PITS serves as a common map or pathway for patient educators. The acronym stands for **P**athophysiology, **I**ndications, **T**reatment, and **S**pecifics. The PITS model was created in an attempt to bring order to patient educational efforts. Order makes a significant difference in the processing and understanding of information (Greenburg, 1991; Ormrod, 2008). The PITS model offers a logical, organized format to deliver health or disease-state information, resulting in a standard communication methodology for the delivery of patient education. In a natural state, PITS flows from disease state toward patient; however, PITS can be inverted to flow information from the patient toward the disease state. An overview of material to be covered should be provided before presenting new information. This helps prepare the receiver for what to expect as the information is presented. Knowing the general trajectory of an educational session can put the learner at ease (Feldman & McPhee, 2008). Delivering the message in digestible bites enhances the receiver's ability to remember the information, as it allows the mental filing of information into related groups or categories (Greenburg, 1991; Ormrod, 2008).

Pathophysiology. Pathology includes all that is physical. The pathology is the segment of education in which the educator identifies any physical changes that have or could occur as the result of a disease, condition, insult, or health state. Physiology refers to biochemical or mechanical changes that occur in the body because of the pathology of the disease or insult. The physiology is the segment of education in which the educator identifies any chemical changes that have occurred or will occur, because of or in relation to the insult or disease process. During this stage of the PITS model a patient learns what is normal and abnormal physically as well as chemically because of the alteration in his health.

As discussed in Section 1, Knowles (1990) asserts that adult learners need to understand "why." Pathophysiology offers the rationale for treatment. Healthcare treatment is ordered to control, prevent, or treat health conditions. All health conditions have a suspected pathophysiologic process for which the healthcare provider formulates actions with the goal of maximizing patient heath. Usually, patients do not have great depth of knowledge regarding pathophysiology, which limits their scope of understanding and their ability to evaluate treatment options beyond their providers' recommendations.

Some argue that the paternalistic nature of healthcare is the result of too much control being assumed by providers, but lack of patient understanding of the "why" associated with suggested treatments may devalue provider recommendations; this could also be a significant factor in poor patient treatment-adherence. A healthcare provider's prescribed recommendations are made based on the provider's expert knowledge of the human body, including a thorough understanding of normal and abnormal bodily functions. Based on the patient's personal report, physical assessment, and diagnostic evaluations, a healthcare provider gathers insight into the patient's health status. The healthcare provider makes educated decisions using this compilation of data. Empirical data, standards of care, and intuition all have a role in guiding providers in the decision-making process, but pathophysiology is the axis on which treatment decisions are ultimately made. Therefore, allowing patients access to this axis may assist patients in making healthcare choices and may directly impact treatment outcomes.

Understanding the pathophysiology also helps establish the association or link between pathophysiology and symptomology or indications of the health status. Recall the discussion of connectionism and the stimulus-response (S-R) model in Chapter 5. Pathophysiology serves as the stimulus for health status indications. Figure 9-1 shows S-R in health teaching.

Stimulus ———————————————————→ **Response**
Health status   *Indications*

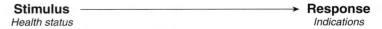

Figure 9-1. Health status and indications related to the stimulus-response model.

Indications. The *I* in PITS represents indications. Indications are the signs or symptoms that may occur as the result of a disease or health state. Symptoms include what the patient may experience as well as what is observed or found on assessment. These symptoms may be used as an indicator of disease progression, maintenance, and/or exacerbation. Explanation of indications occurs during this step of the PITS model. The educator should start by reviewing the previously covered material from the P step, pathophysiology, including physical and chemical changes. Correlating the physical or chemical changes with the related symptoms can help the patient better relate to his health status and sets the foundation for treatment choices. By teaching the pathophysiology followed by an explanation of indications, the educator is progressively building patient knowledge in blocks of information. Each block of information adds to and builds on the previous block. The pathophysiology should serve as the stimulus for the response that occurs in indications, as seen in Figure 9-2.

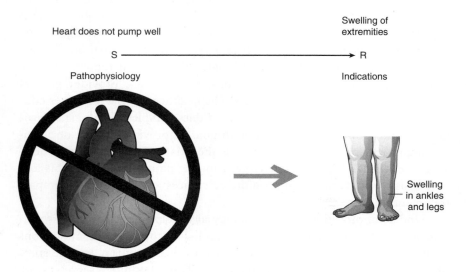

Figure 9-2. The illustration relates pathophysiology and indications to the stimulus-response model in the example of congestive heart failure.

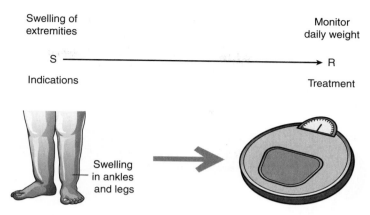

Figure 9-3. The illustration relates indications and treatment to the stimulus-response model in the example of congestive heart failure.

Once the P and I steps are covered, the patient should have a beginning understanding of the provider's view, which directly influences provider decisions and treatment course choices. Redman (2007) asserts that patients need a rationale for ordered treatment, especially when behavior change is involved. The *PI* of PITS serves as the rationale for the reason a treatment is ordered. Figure 9-3 represents the S-R relationship of the indications and treatment stages of the PITS model.

Treatment. Treatment is the gold standard or the industry-accepted industry to managing or resolving the disease or health state for which the provider is treating the patient. In this stage, treatment information specific to the disease or health state is provided. Complex instructions need to be broken down and taught one step at a time. This may include information about how to administer insulin for insulin-dependent diabetics, or daily weight monitoring for congestive heart failure patients as shown in Figure 9-3. Pamphlets, handouts, videos, and other such educational tools can be used for this stage because the information is not specific to the patient. As in previous steps, it is useful here to go back and build on the information covered in the P and I steps. Reviewing previous steps provides insight into "why" the behavior or treatment is being suggested. Each step of PITS continues to build on the previous step. Repetition of previous steps will reinforce information through conditioning or strengthening associations through the law of exercise (Lefrancois, 1995; Thorndike, 1932), as

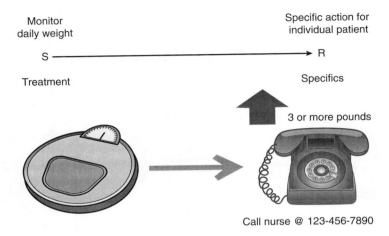

Figure 9-4. The illustration relates the treatment and specifics to the stimulus-response model for congestive heart failure.

well as help to organize the mental connection of new information with present schema (Anderson, Spiro, & Montague, 1984; Armbruster, 1996; Ormrod, 2008; Shuell, 1990). The repetition of previously reviewed content helps move information along through the three stages of memory noted in Chapter 5 (Balota & Marsh 2004).

Specifics. Up to this point, information has been mostly disease or health-state centered. As patient education moves to the final step of PITS, specifics, the information becomes patient-centered. In this step, the information delivered is tailored specifically for each patient, hence, patient-specific instruction. During the S step, personal medications with individual dosages, diet restrictions specifically designed for the patient, and individual activity restrictions are reviewed. This stage cannot be taught to a classroom of patients; this stage is only about one individual—the patient.

Like every stage before, reviewing information from the previous steps helps the patient process the material in an orderly and sequential manner. Previous steps should provide a logical foundation for the information that is covered in this stage. Figure 9-4 illustrates the presence of S-R as information transitions from the T step to the S step of PITS.

PITS Model in Action. PITS serves as a guide for health-material delivery. Patients need to better understand their disease processes in order to

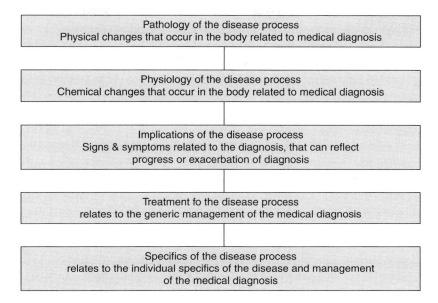

Figure 9-5. A brief outline of the PITS model, including an explanation of the meaning and focus for each step.

participate in their care and be more than just recipients of care. The PITS model follows the diagnosis and treatment process (Figure 9-5). For example, a patient presents with symptoms (indications), the patient is assessed (pathology), lab work is done (physiology), and treatment is ordered (standards of practice) reflecting specifics of individualized needs (personalized individualized care ordered and information needed). PITS serves as a way of communicating with the healthcare consumer throughout the diagnosis, planning, treatment, and maintenance phases of care. The PITS model provides an outline of what, how, and why for the patient, then offers generalized solutions followed by specific solutions. The PITS model serves to define a pathway healthcare providers can use to deliver information as they guide healthcare consumers toward their personal healthcare goals.

PITS is not specific to a particular discipline and can be used by any healthcare provider. It is recommended that healthcare providers review each step in the order of the model even if the intent is to teach information in the last step.

Case Study

Haddie, the retired cafeteria worker from Chapter 8, needs to learn about her chronic illness—congestive heart failure. The nurse needs to teach Haddie weight-parameter triggers for calling the provider along with the phone number to call. The nurse begins her instruction with a brief review of pathophysiology and indications: "Remember how when the heart is not pumping effectively (pathophysiology) the body will hold water and may swell (indications)? Daily weights (treatment) are needed to help identify when the body is holding water before there is a lot of swelling. If you experience a three-pound or greater weight gain in your morning weight, you will need to call your nurse at this number (specifics)."

The physical therapist needs to teach the same patient about safe ambulation. The physical therapist reviews pathophysiology and indications first: "Remember your heart pump is not effectively working (pathophysiology) so the body may hold water or swell (indications)." He goes on to cover daily weights (traditional treatment) and its use in identifying when the body is holding water before there is too much swelling. He tells Haddie that she will need to use her walker as she goes to weigh in the morning (specifics). He instructs Haddie on how to position the scale so the walker can move over the scale. Once on the scale, the therapist tells Haddie to hold onto the walker until she is balanced. When balanced he advises her to look at the number then let go, look at number again, then re-grip the walker. He estimates that she should not have to let her walker go for more than a minute. This example demonstrates how two separate disciplines can teach the same patient using PITS. Figure 9-6 displays the progression of information using PITS in two different disciplines.

The revisiting of each step previously covered in PITS serves as a foundation for progression to the next step, assisting the receiver in the accommodation and assimilation of the new information (Lund, Carruth, Moody, & Logan, 2005; Novak, 1998; Saunders, 1992). Perpetually revisiting information provides reinforcement of the information, which helps to mentally "stamp in" knowledge and move new data into the long-term memory (Cowan, 2001; MacGregor, 1987; Thorndike, 1932). Providers

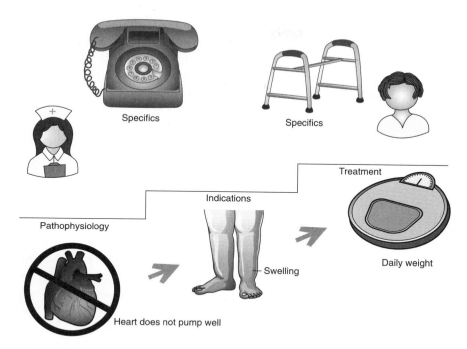

Figure 9-6. The combined steps of PITS from the perspectives of two different disciplines. The PIT—pathophysiology, indication, and treatment—steps provide the foundation for the specific exercises the physical therapist wants the patient to do, and also supports the call the nurse wants the patient to make regarding specific changes in daily weights.

deliver treatment information and specifics framed by the focus of their discipline. For example, nursing may focus on self-care teaching, a dietitian may focus on diet teaching, the doctor may discuss diagnostics needed, the physical therapist may focus on mobility safety and exercise, while the pharmacist focuses on medication administration. When the information is presented by multiple disciplines in the same manner, it shows patients that their providers are unified in their approach while offering the benefit of reinforcing information. Empowering patients with information elevates consumers to partners, and gives them a degree of responsibility in their healthcare.

The first two steps of PITS, pathophysiology and indications, should not vary by discipline. The treatment step is where the variation may begin according to the focus of each provider's discipline. For example, a physical therapist treating a patient who has received PI instruction would briefly review pathophysiology and indications, then focus on the exercises ordered. The physical therapist may pull from the pathology and indications to correlate the exercises relevant to the symptoms experienced, or to the disease pathology and how the exercises will decrease the problems experienced, or improve physical alterations. This gives meaning and justification to the exercises. It also helps give the patient direct control in achieving optimal health. The patient can directly correlate an activity to improvement in his health conditions. The number of exercise sets or repetitions, as well as any alterations personalized for the patient, moves the therapist teaching into the specifics stage.

Evaluation of presenting knowledge is easier if the patient's healthcare providers are using PITS. The provider simply needs to evaluate the patient's understanding of each step to see where the patient is in his knowledge. A noticeable deficit in one step should alert providers to concentrate their efforts on that information step. PITS offers a universal teaching model for all disease processes and for all disciplines. Whether physician, therapist, dietitian, or nurse, all disciplines can follow PITS, each adding to the patient's treatment. Each provider focuses on the same disease, treating and teaching from his or her discipline and building on the patient education efforts of their colleagues while improving their patient's health knowledge. Providers may never meet, but by using the same model they build on each other's educational contributions.

SUMMARY

- Information needs to flow logically so it can be easily received, filed, and retrieved by the recipient.

- Information delivered in an orderly fashion makes sense and allows the receiver to easily follow the educator's train of thought.

- Complex instructions need to be broken down and taught one step at a time.

- Redman (2007) points out that information needs to be delivered in an orderly, sequential style according to the patient's order of need. Information should flow either from disease toward the patient or away from the patient toward disease.

- The PITS model was created in an attempt to bring order to patient educational efforts. It offers a logical, organized format to deliver health or disease-state information, resulting in a standard communication methodology for the delivery of patient education. In a natural state, PITS flows from disease state toward patient; however, it can be inverted to flow information from the patient toward the disease state.

- PITS is an acronym that serves as a patient education model, a common map or pathway for patient education. The acronym stands for pathophysiology, indications, treatment, and specifics.

- The *P* denotes pathophysiology. Pathology includes all that is physical. The pathology is the segment of education in which the educator identifies any physical changes that have occurred or could occur as the result of a disease, condition, insult, or health state.

- The *I* in PITS represents indications. Indications are the signs or symptoms that may occur as the result of the disease or health state. Symptoms include what the patient may experience as well as what may be observed or found on assessment. These symptoms may be used as an indicator of disease progression, maintenance, and exacerbation.

- The *PI* of PITS serves as the rationale for the reason a treatment is ordered.

- The *T* of PITS refers to treatment. Treatment is the gold standard or industry-accepted approach to managing or resolving the disease or health state for which the provider is treating the patient. In this stage, treatment information specific to the disease or health state is provided.

- The *S* refers to specifics. This is the personalization of treatment. In this stage, the information delivered is tailored specifically for that patient, hence, patient-specific instruction. During this stage, personal medications with individual dosages, diet restrictions only for that patient, and individual activity restrictions are reviewed.

- The PITS model provides an outline of what, how, and why for the patient, then offers generalized solutions followed by specific solutions. The model defines a pathway healthcare providers can use to deliver information as they guide healthcare consumers toward their personal healthcare goals.

- PITS is not specific to a particular discipline and can be used by any healthcare provider. It is recommended that healthcare providers review each step in the order of the model even if the intent is to teach information in the last step.

- The revisiting of each stage previously covered in PITS serves as a foundation for progression to the next stage, assisting the receiver in the accommodation and assimilation of the new information.

- The first two steps of PITS, pathophysiology and indications, should not vary by discipline. The treatment stage is where the variation may begin according to the focus of the discipline.

- Each provider focuses on the same disease, treating and teaching from his or her discipline and building on the patient education efforts of their colleagues while improving their patients' health knowledge. Providers may never meet, but by using the same model they build on each other's educational contributions.

[CHAPTER 10]

The Medagogy Conceptual Framework

In healthcare, the provider and the patient should share one guiding common interest: the patient's health. The patient should be the focus of all decisions. All interactions and treatment should be predicated on respect for patients including their ability and right to know and understand their healthcare treatment, choices, obligations, and commitments. The hope is that healthcare providers are able to meet patients' needs and help patients reach or exceed their personal health goals.

In order to accomplish this, there must be effective communication between provider and patient as well as between providers. The PITS model discussed in Chapter 9 offers a common pathway for information delivery, exchange, flow, processing, and influence in the decision-making process. The medagogy conceptual framework focuses on the overarching process of patient education while concentrating on the flow and operation of information. This theoretical structure includes the steps of health knowledge gain, the informational seasons of patient education, and the PITS model. This conceptual philosophy is meant to serve as a common framework for information delivery in the daily practice of patient education. Medagogy succinctly communicates the complexities of patient education in healthcare. Figure 10-1 displays the medagogy Conceptual Framework.

The beauty of this theoretical framework lies in the unlimited possibilities provided by the individual's values and interpretations. However, that great variety also creates a problem when the time comes to implement the conceptual framework. If medagogy is to serve as a common model for a team, then all members of the team need to have a working knowledge

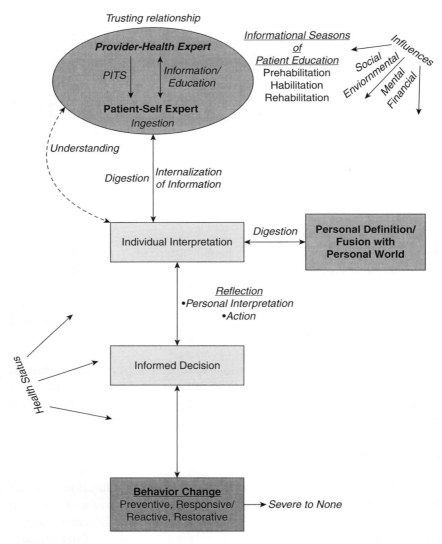

Figure 10-1. In the medagogy Conceptual Framework, the flow of information in patient education is displayed as all of the components of patient education are pulled together, from the patient-provider relationship, through internalization of information, to the ultimate behavior changes that result from informed decision making.

of the model and its impact on practice. Just as patients need time to ingest, digest, and reflect on information, the same is true for members of the healthcare team. Once information has been self-interpreted and action ensues, then team members can decide how to put the model into practice as a team.

INFORMATION MOVEMENT IN MEDAGOGY

The medagogy model provides definition to the process of patient learning by identifying the components of information-exchange in the patient education process. Medagogy maintains that patient learning begins with a trusting relationship between healthcare provider and patient. In the provider-patient relationship, the provider serves as the expert of health and the patient serves as the expert of self. A certain level of power comes with expert status.

Healthcare providers have long been comfortable with the power associated with expert status (Shea, 2006). Medagogy asserts that no other person can know more about self than self. Therefore, in the patient-provider relationship, the patient must assume the rightful position as expert of self.

Information flow is continuous between provider and patient. Information exchanged ranges from exposure to instruction, and may contain any material from personal facts and data to casual lighthearted dialogue. Treatment directions and suggestions should be formatted so that patients can understand the information, make informed decisions, and follow through with established health plans.

The information exchanged by the patient and the provider is internalized by each. As the internalized information is assimilated, an individual interpretation evolves. With the addition of new information to the patient's personal knowledge base, individual interpretation merges the newly acquired information with the patient's personal world. Once the information is integrated into the patient's personal world, it can be accessed as needed for everyday living. The resulting interpretation helps guide the patient's decision-making process. The same is true for the provider; understanding the unique aspects of a patient enhances the provider's ability to make informed and personalized decisions.

Information reception, processing and decision-making is affected by the patient's health status and other influences like physical, mental, financial, environmental, and social status along with cultural and spiritual beliefs (Falvo, 1994; Henderson, 2002; Pierce & Hicks, 2001; Prossier, Almond, & Walley, 2003; Stewart, Meredith, Brown, & Galajda, 2000). Physical phenomena include physical limitations like motor control or ability, vision, hearing, tolerance, and comfort (Stewart, Meredith, Brown, & Galajda, 2000). Mental activity influences include learning disabilities, cognitive deficit, and illness or treatment haze where mental clarity is hazy secondary to illness or treatment, as in the cases of surgery recovery or pain-medication usage (Falvo, 1994; Stewart, Meredith, Brown, & Galajda, 2000). Financial influences include financial obligations, limitations, and constraints (Greene & Adelman, 2003; Henderson, 2002). Environmental influences are related to the physical environment of the healthcare setting, personal home, work, and social surroundings (Curtis, Patrick, Caldwell, & Collier, 2000; Falvo, 1994; Gabbay, Cowie, Kerr, & Purdy, 2000). Social influences include social networks, community, culture, and the attitudes of family and friends, in addition to accepted and adopted norms (Kravitz et al., 2002). Spiritual influences include personal, cultural, and faith-based beliefs and values (Falvo, 1994; Greene & Adelman, 2003).

Certified Patient Educators (CPEs) offer invaluable expertise to the healthcare team that is committed to addressing patient literacy in their practice. The CPE played an integral role in the success of the Centers for Medicare and Medicaid System's (CMS) care transitions pilot as mentioned previously. In the care transitions pilot, the CPEs initiated a structured patient education plan for each patient that was accepted into the Louisiana project. They managed a population of patients' knowledge needs as patients safely transitioned from acute (dependent care) to home (self/independent care) and assisted patients to successfully meet their treatment plan goals, inclusive of follow-up healthcare access. Together the CPEs and their extender, the Patient Specialist (PS-c), helped their patients avoid readmission and inappropriate resource utilization.

A CPE can be requested to evaluate a patient, or a protocol can require all admitted patients to be evaluated by a CPE. Evaluation needs to include the patient's learning style (primary and secondary), ideal time of day for learning, admitting level of knowledge, learning disabilities, need for learning aides, and the patient's perception of his learning needs. Working within the trusting relationship, identified in the conceptual model for medagogy, the patient educator—as an expert of health— exchanges information with the patient, who is recognized as the expert of

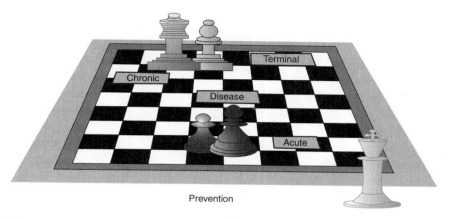

Figure 10-2. The illustration displays the personal positioning of individuals with regard to their health throughout life.

self. The informational seasons discussed in Chapter 7 help the CPE deliver information according to the patient's health positioning. Figure 10-2 represents positioning of health in life. After assessment and information exchange, the CPE can draft a teaching plan that includes learning objectives, teaching materials to be used, methods of instruction, and modes of evaluating comprehension, and aligns team members' contributions.

After the teaching plan is drafted, it can then serve as a form of communication between providers regarding the patient's progress toward health knowledge. The teaching plan transitions into a report card system that can flow between providers as each one contributes to the plan. The report-card system serves as a tool to communicate progress, but also contains an assessment of the patient's learning needs. With a quick glance, each provider can determine how best to deliver information to the patient. The report card also provides insight into the patient's strengths and weaknesses regarding knowledge. The report card should be a never-ending, living document that follows the patient throughout the healthcare system. As patients transition between providers and care settings, they are exposed to copious health-sustaining information that is often lost, misunderstood, or undervalued. Just as physical care alterations are exchanged between healthcare settings and healthcare providers, patient health knowledge should also progress through the system with the patient. New objectives and teaching methods are added as the patient's knowledge and/

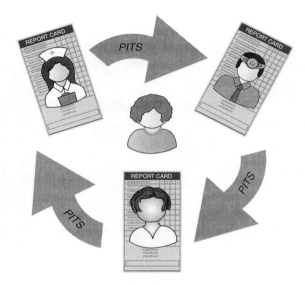

Figure 10-3. Information exchange between providers is accomplished by using a report card system. The patient and the CPE serve as a hub for the patient's present level of understanding and progression of knowledge.

or health status changes. Figure 10-3 displays the report-card exchange as it moves through various providers.

The CPE or designated patient educator can periodically evaluate the patient's comprehension to provide a common, consistent provider evaluation. In addition, learning boosters or refreshers from occasional educational sessions can help a patient who is not actively engaged in healthcare delivery continue to avoid the need to access healthcare because of acute episodic symptomology. By refreshing the patient's memory with previously reviewed information, previously stored information can be reactivated and information that may not have made it into long-term memory can work through the stages of memory. Re-exposure to information helps to re-energize stored information (Zull, 2006). It is easier to re-learn information forgotten or not retained (Sousa, 2006). The booster provides a mental boost of information for the patient so that information does not become stagnant or stale, which may lead to nonuse of information and/or decreased exactness of the information (Feldman & McPhee, 2008; Ormrod, 2008). Engaging patients when they are not in a crisis or an acute health situation helps to re-energize the neural forests discussed in Chapter 8 and awaken patients' consciousness of their health while, hopefully, providing a less emotionally challenging teaching opportunity (Zull, 2006).

INGESTION TO DIGESTION

Once information is received or ingested, the breakdown of the information, or mental digestion, begins. Digestion in the gastrointestinal system of the body involves the chemical and physical breakdown of ingested food. The food is separated, then stored or discarded according to how the body will need or use it. The mental ingestion and digestion of information is very similar to the gastrointestinal process. Information received is internalized, or taken in, through ingestion. In the digestion of information, personal values and beliefs help in the personal interpretation of information. Who, how, when, and where all play a part in influencing personal perception of information.

Personal definition involves individual values and beliefs along with personal world, which includes social support systems and social interactions like family, friends, and job. In the book *Through the Patient's Eyes,* attention is drawn to the need for healthcare providers to be respectful of patients' life experiences, culture, and beliefs, including the impacts of these on healthcare decision-making (Gerteis et al., 1993). Medagogy attempts to capture the effect of individualism in the medagogic process of interpretation resulting from fusion of new information with the personal world. Personal world is a conglomeration of all the intricacies of personal life, including recreational activities like exercise and hobbies, as well as faith-based convictions and political practices. Fishbein and Ajzen (1975) acknowledge in their predictive persuasion theory, discussed in Chapter 6, that personal beliefs influence a person's behavior. Pender and colleagues (2002) capture medagogy's concept of the personal world in their health promotion model as interpersonal influences. If something is important enough for the patient to participate in regularly, it is of value to the patient. Even if participation is a requirement of a relationship, the follow-through of participation is representative of worth. The worth of participation may be based in the value of the relationship.

Case Study

Laurie, a professor at the local college, and her husband Jim, a local plumber, faithfully attend all of the local college's football games. Laurie does not like football, but the event is not the impetus of her action. The relationship with her spouse is where the value lies. So why would this be important in health? Health can impact how people live life. The better patients feel, the more they are able to live life without unhealthy inhibition. Health can divert personal life temporarily or permanently. For example, the acute and temporary health change of a broken leg may make attendance at football games impossible for the remainder of the season. Whereas, a diagnosis of muscular dystrophy may gradually decrease the physical stamina required for football game attendance as a permanent and chronic health alteration. Health behavior choices are influenced by individual interpretation, which is perpetually affected by one's personal world.

Individuals do not determine the value of all information internally. Some information is deemed of personal worth in concert with external influences at the time of ingestion, digestion, and reflection. Health status is a major external influence on the patient's mental processing of information. Health status reflects where patients are on their health continuum. A fever with head congestion may influence the ingestion of information. The congestion may decrease the ability to hear what is being said, while the fever may cause a distracted mentality that could influence the processing of information. Medications and health indications can decrease alertness, affecting the abilities to mentally file information and successfully move through the stages of memory (short- to long-term). Health status also refers to Bishop's (1991) suggestion that patients make their own mental representation of any alteration in health. Simpson and colleagues (1991) discuss the variance in perceptions between provider and patient, including illness perceptions. Part of the disparity is related to varying illness representations, which can be attributed to individualism as well as internal and external influences like health (Skevington & Garro, 1995; Weinman, Petrie & Moss-Morris, 1996).

Environmental influences relate to the physical environment of the healthcare setting and the person's home, work, and social surroundings. When educating the patient, the environment where the patient is taught can influence learning (Falvo, 1994; Redman, 2007). A patient educator can evaluate physical surroundings using his senses: visual, auditory, tactile, taste, and even smell. The setting in which the healthcare information is delivered might be noisy, with competing sounds that interfere with receiving information. The setting may contain visual distractions, making it difficult for the patient to focus on the message. Senses like touch, taste, and smell bear mentioning because they have influencing power. The sense of touch determines if the environment is comfortable; consider the room's physical temperature or seating, as well as the general physical comfort of the patient. The sense of smell can physically impact a person. For example, noxious smells can be distracting, while some aromas can be stimulating and make a person more receptive to learning. Some treatments can cause a bad taste in the mouth, which can be a negative distraction. Environment may also include conditions like the provider-patient relationship. The provider-patient relationship can be influenced by a patient's desire to please the provider; it can also cause dissatisfaction and distrust in a patient (Heisler, Bouknight, Hayward, & Smith, 2002). The environmental influence of the provider's healthcare decision-making style will determine if the provider is open to patient inclusion in the treatment planning process (Guadagnoli & Ward, 1998; Van de Borne, 1998). A cooperative partnership environment will encourage and support patient involvement in making healthcare decisions (Guadagnoli & Ward, 1998).

Fishbein and Ajzen's (1975) predictive persuasion theory accounts for the social environment's influence on a person's behavior. Medagogy also acknowledges the impact that social influence may have on patient health decisions and, ultimately, patient actions. Social influence is so important that it is captured both in internal and external influences. Beyond the internal composition of one's personal world as an external influence, social influences include cultural and social networks, community, the attitudes of family and friends, as well as accepted and adopted norms.

Medagogy attempts to determine social influences of which the patient may not even be aware. External social influences may occur through subconscious conditioning (as discussed under Behaviorism in Chapter 5) via social norms that have meshed with self over time.

Case Study

External social influence is noted in the following example of assumed passivity in the patient role. Like many people Bob, an ex-Marine, was told to take his medicine when he was a child. He was also told to be quiet when the doctors, as well as other adults, were talking. Young Bob went to the doctor for boosters, vaccinations, and when he was not feeling well. Over time, Bob was conditioned to dread doctor visits and to passively follow doctors' advice without question. Not all people assume the level of passivity that Bob acquired over time. Bob internalized and accepted certain social influences as a child; Bob's passivity in the patient role is a lingering bias he still carries in his adulthood. Bob's decisions in his healthcare will be made in the presence of this personal bias.

External mental influence is captured as presenting knowledge and the ability to acquire knowledge. Presenting knowledge may be in any subject matter, including but not limited to health. As discussed in Bloom's taxonomy in Chapter 5, is the patient able to create or do they remember? The ability to acquire knowledge involves the patient's learning style and preferences, including capabilities and limitations, as well as the patient's circadian rhythm for learning. For example, is the patient a morning learner or an evening learner? Learning capabilities and limitations include learning disabilities, history of learning successes and failures, cognitive deficit, and illness or treatment haze affecting mental clarity (such as surgery recovery or pain-medication usage). Refer to Chapter 5 for a detailed discussion of learning styles.

Financial influences like financial obligations, limitations, and constraints are also external influences. Financial influences can be profoundly distracting for a patient. A patient's concern about treatment cost can induce feelings of fear and anxiety, which can impact patient decision making. Financial impact can also limit treatment choices because of a patient's personal financial constraints. Piette and colleagues (2004) surveyed 660 Americans about medication cost. Survey findings revealed that 440 of those surveyed confessed that they underuse their prescribed medications because of cost and they have never told their healthcare provider. Interestingly, 435 of the survey respondents also reported that they have never been asked if they can afford their prescribed medication (Piette, Heisler, & Wagner, 2004). Another financial concern well documented in the literature is the healthcare provider's personal financial gain related to the prescribed treatment, pointing to the question of patient versus personal interests affecting treatment decisions (Emaneul & Goldman, 1998; Levinson et al., 1999).

 Case Study

John, a 64-year-old male patient, is a local businessman and needs a kidney transplant. John does not have health insurance and cannot afford to pay for the organ transplant. John's financial status limits his treatment options and excludes the transplant option from his menu of treatment choices.

Reflection of knowledge begins to become apparent in the transition from personal interpretation to informed decision. All of the previous factors and their influencing powers are present in the informed decision. The degree to which they are acknowledged or used is personal, but their presence is there. The presence of these other factors offers insight into why the patient should have an understanding of the information influencing the healthcare provider's treatment decisions. Without their providers' information about pathophysiology, indications, textbook treatment, and individual specifics, patients can rely only on what they already know. Not knowing the pathophysiology, indications, textbook treatment, and individual specifics limits the patient's ability to make an informed decision. Knowing these things balances the decision with health knowledge.

 Case Study

Lulu, a local housewife, has no knowledge about how cars work. She brings her car to a shop because it has been making a strange noise. The mechanic queries her, then looks at the engine and the underside of the car. The mechanic tells Lulu that she will need a $2000 engine repair. Lulu asks

"Why?" The mechanic replies, "Because the car engine is sick." Lulu then asks for an explanation. The mechanic explains the problem with the car using mechanical terminology like chassis, head gasket, crankshaft, and cylinder head. The mechanic hears a bell, signaling the next client's arrival and hurriedly tells the woman, "You just think about it and let me know what you decide." Before he can leave her, Lulu asks, "What will happen if I do not do the work you recommend?" The mechanic responds, "The car will die," as he hands her a bill and tells her to pay the lady at the window on her way out, then walks away. Dazed and confused, Lulu immediately tries to call her best friend to get advice as she makes her way to the payment window. Lulu's best friend tells her not to worry, that her sister's car did the same thing and it just went away. She advises Lulu to forget about it and not to let the mechanic take advantage of her. Lulu takes her best friend's advice and the car stalls just two blocks from the mechanic's shop. Mechanical knowledge of the problem could have helped Lulu balance her decision-making with knowledge she unaware of, the information the mechanic was using to make his mechanical diagnosis.

Decisions that patients make reflect their interpretation of the situation, values, influencing factors, and understanding. If the decision is made with accurate understanding of the pathophysiology of the health status, indications, treatment, and specifics, then the patient has made an informed decision. Action occurs based on the patient's decision. Medagogy focuses on the action of behavior change. Behavior change may be severe, such as a complete change from presenting behavior and lifestyle. For example, consider a cardiac, overweight, and sedentary person who decides to diet and exercise daily to improve his heart-health. No change would mean the cardiac patient decides not to make any lifestyle changes, including medication administration. No change in behavior is still considered an action because it is represents choice. Whatever the patient's decision, as long as the provider has made health information available and understandable to the patient, then the healthcare provider should respect the patient's choice. The healthcare provider should always make the information that they are using to guide health treatment decisions available to the patient even if the patient has chosen not to change behavior.

Behavior change that does occur in response to informed decision may be preventive, responsive or reactive, or restorative. These behavior changes are reflective of the patient's informational season (see

Chapter 7). The prehabilitative informational season of patient education, involves the delivery of information to a patient at risk for an insult
to health. The behavior change that is associated with this informational
season is prevention. Preventive behavior change occurs prior to an insult
to health. The focus of prevention is to avoid negative health status. The
goal is for prehabilitative education to yield preventive behavior change
in the patient. Once an insult to health has occurred, the patient then
enters the habilitation informational season. In habilitation, the information is focused on developing new lifestyle habits to help control health
status and avoid negative health outcomes. Responsive or reactive behavior change occurs in response to a negative change in health status. The
behavior change is warranted to control, or to try to control, the health
state. The rehabilitation informational season focuses educational efforts
on helping the patient regain any loss that has occurred as the result of
negative health status. Restorative behavior change occurs in response to
a negative health occurrence. Behavior is focused on restoring health to a
pre-insult health state. Figure 10-4 displays the relationship of the informational seasons to patient behavior change.

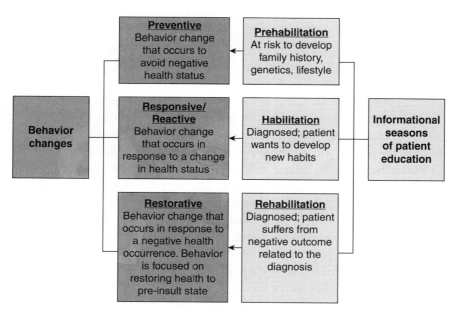

Figure 10-4.   The informational seasons of patient education are related to the types
of behavior changes they can produce.

Medagogy serves as a model to connect all of the elements of the patient education process, from information delivery to action. Medagogy views informational processing in patient education from the patient's perspective.

Medagogy's conceptual framework begins with the initial exchange between two experts—provider, the expert of health, and patient, the expert of self—through the internalization of information. Informational seasons of patient education help orient information to a patient's present health status in relation to health concerns identified by the healthcare provider. Information delivered to the patient initiates movement toward acquiring health knowledge. Along the path of gaining knowledge, internal and external personal influences are encountered as the patient begins to merge the health state with self. The individualism of understanding is revealed in reflection, where action occurs based on the patient's informed decision. The medagogy model attempts to communicate the many facets involved in patients' processing of provided information and the impacts of their perceptions on decision making.

CONSTRUCTING INFORMATION FOR DELIVERY TO PATIENTS

Once a patient's learning styles and preferences are identified, they should become part of the patient's health demographic information. As a provider plans to educate a patient, he should reference the patient's education hierarchy as well as the informational seasons of patient education (see Chapter 7). After the patient's informational season and level on the hierarchy are identified, the patient educator needs to choose a method of delivery for patient information. Prior to information delivery, the method for evaluating patient understanding should be identified. Once these key pieces are in place education can begin. The purpose of the teaching intervention should be clear to both patient and provider prior to initiation so that a level of achievement can be determined.

Medagogy offers a glimpse into the patient's learning process versus traditional healthcare initiatives that are more provider-centered, focusing on what will be delivered and when it will be delivered. Instead of working the patient into healthcare provider plans, medagogy invites providers to step back and move with the patient rather than being two steps ahead of them. This is not to say the medagogy model must be utilized independently.

As evidenced in the CMS care transitions pilot, medagogy can complement successful projects like RED (Reengineering Hospital Discharge) and BOOST (Better Outcomes for Older Adults through Safe Transitions) beautifully. Either project can be implemented with medagogy concepts to help providers deliver patient-centered communication while harnessing the full power of individual patient education efforts. Interdependently and/or independently, medagogy can assist providers as they help their patients gain physical and mental control of their health.

SUMMARY

- In healthcare, the provider and the patient should both share one guiding common interest: the patient's health. The patient should be the focus of all decisions.

- In order to accomplish this, there must be effective communication between provider and patient as well as between providers. The PITS model offers a common pathway for information delivery, exchange, flow, processing, and influence in the decision-making process.

- If medagogy is to serve as a common model for a team, then all members of the team need to have a working knowledge of the model and its impact on practice.

- Certified Patient Educators (CPEs) offer invaluable expertise to the healthcare team that is committed to addressing patient literacy in their practice.

- After assessment and information exchange, the patient educator can begin to draft a teaching plan including learning objectives, teaching materials to be used, methods of instruction, modes of evaluation of comprehension, and names of responsible providers.

- After the teaching plan is drafted, it can serve as a form of communication between providers regarding the patient's progress toward health knowledge.

- A CPE or designated patient educator can periodically do evaluations of comprehension to provide a common, consistent provider evaluation.

- Once information is received or ingested, the breakdown of the information or mental digestion begins. The mental ingestion and digestion of information is very similar to the gastrointestinal process. Information received is internalized, or taken in, through ingestion.

- When educating the patient, the environment where the patient is taught can influence learning. A patient educator can evaluate physical surroundings using his own senses: visual, auditory, tactile, taste, and even smell.

- Environment may include the condition of the provider-patient relationship. The provider-patient relationship can be influenced by a patient's desire to please the provider; it can also cause dissatisfaction and distrust in a patient.

- Financial influences like financial obligations, limitations, and constraints are considered external influences. Financial influences can be profoundly distracting for a patient.

- Not knowing the pathophysiology, indications, textbook treatment, and individual specifics limits the patient's ability to make an informed decision. Knowing these things balances the decision with health knowledge.

- The decisions that patients make are a reflection of their interpretation of the situation, values, influencing factors, and understanding.

- Whatever a patient's decision, as long as the provider has made health information available and understandable to the patient, then the healthcare provider should respect the patient's choice.

- Behavior change that occurs in response to informed decision may be preventive, responsive or reactive, or restorative.

- The medagogy model serves to connect all of the elements in the patient education process, from information delivery to action. Medagogy views informational processing in patient education from the patient's perspective.

- Medagogy's conceptual framework begins with the initial exchange between two experts—provider, the expert of health, and patient, the expert of self—through the internalization of information.

- Once patients' learning styles and preferences are identified, they should become part of their health demographic information.

- The purpose of the teaching intervention should be clear to both patient and provider prior to initiation so level of achievement can be determined.

- Medagogy can complement successful projects such as RED (Reengineering Hospital Discharge) and BOOST (Better Outcomes for Older Adults through Safe Transitions).

[CHAPTER 11]

The UPP Tool: Assessing Patient Knowledge

As healthcare becomes more patient oriented, providers will have to treat each patient as an individual. The aspiration of a new patient-oriented community of care can only become reality by addressing each patient's health literacy needs. Through a structured approach to patient education and communication, providers can unite their efforts and progressively add to each individual patient's health knowledge reservoir.

The Institute of Medicine's (IOM's) (2004) report has suggested that all health professions engage in program activities that emphasize respect for and understanding of cultural and individual patient and family diversity (Smedley, Butler, & Bristow, 2004). The IOM further emphasizes that personal and demographic characteristics such as age, disability, ethnicity, gender, language, national origin, religion, sexual orientation, and socio-economic status be considered when planning all aspects of patient care. Importantly, this approach must also include patient education. The medagogy model emphasizes cultural and individual diversity and reinforces the assumption that every human being is uniquely different (M. Jewell, personal communication, March 10, 2010).

The medagogy framework offers a pathway for educating individuals that can be beneficial in chronic illness management and care coordination. Treatment and management of chronic illness translates financially into more than 1 trillion dollars of the annual U.S. federal healthcare budget (Wagner, 2004). It is imperative that self-care and self-management be buttressed in all patient education teachings, especially for those individuals with chronic health conditions. According to Wagner (2004), 95% of Medicare's budget is spent on chronic illness. Two-thirds of the 65-years-of-age and older population lives with four or more chronic health conditions; prevention along with improved self-care and self-management can help preserve our nation's limited healthcare resources, both human and fiscal (Wagner, 2004). A healthier nation of people due to informed engagement in self-care is a realistic and noble goal.

KNOWLEDGE MEASUREMENT

Patient education should include evaluative techniques to assess patient understanding (Redman, 2003). Historically, standard knowledge measurement that is traditional to academic settings has not been used in healthcare. Tests and quizzes and performance-based assessments of knowledge are not a common practice in patient education (Falvo, 1994; Lainscak & Keber, 2005; Redman, 2001; 2003). Instead, in patient education a loose qualitative labeling suffices as the "norm" for knowledge evaluation (Escalante, et al., 2004; Freeman & Chambers, 1997). For instance, if a patient is exposed to health information, the healthcare provider may document "able to verbalize understanding" or "able to repeat back" (Escalante, et al., 2004; Freeman & Chambers, 1997). Neither of these examples offers insight as to where the patient is in their knowledge attainment. The first example "able to verbalize understanding" could possibly even be a brush-off from the patient like "of course, I got it." The second example, "able to repeat back," is commonly seen in exotic birds and parrots, which is why parroting is a fitting label for this sort of appraisal. Neither example hits the mark of identifying the patient's status in learning, nor does either example give the healthcare provider the ability to understand a patient's grasp of information.

Providers need a systematic approach to use in evaluating and following a patient's knowledge gain as they strive to move patients toward greater health awareness and independence. Vague and limited provider insight, at best, is achieved through present patient education evaluation methods. Capturing the progression of patient knowledge and intervening when knowledge deficits put the patient at risk can help the patient avoid unnecessary health setbacks as well as inappropriate or avoidable resource utilization. Perpetually increasing the patient's knowledge as he moves throughout the healthcare system will advance the patient toward independent self-care, health sustainability, and health autonomy.

NEED FOR A PATIENT PERCEPTION TOOL

Universally, health literacy definitions acknowledge patients' needs to understand and utilize health information to which they have been exposed. Feldman and McPhee (2008) acknowledge that comprehension and understanding are abstract; therefore, direct measurement is often challenging. Although instruments serve as a form of assessment to determine the level of understanding of a subject or content, results can be misleading. Fears, poor test-taking skills, low reading literacy, the quality of items on the measurement tools or instruments, and sometimes poorly selected variables can affect test results. The results could misrepresent a person's understanding of information which translates, in clinical practice, to insufficient self-care information.

To determine the state of the science, Stewart conducted a literature review which revealed that a number of measures have been developed to assess patient knowledge. The Michigan Diabetes Research Training Centers (MDRTC) diabetes knowledge test consists of 23 multiple-choice questions (Fitzgerald et al., 1998; Redman, 2003). Approximately 15 minutes is required to complete the MDTRC knowledge test (Redman, 2003). Reliabilty and validity was first collected in a study of 811 participants from two different Michigan communities; one community received at-home services for their diabetes care (312 subjects), while the second community received diabetes care in a Michigan Department of Public Health clinical setting (499 subjects). The two sample populations were similar in diabetes type, treatment, years since diagnosis, and academic education completed. The populations varied in age, gender, ethnicity, and previous diabetic education. The public health clinic population included fewer Caucasians, more females, younger participants, and fewer subjects having received previous diabetic education. Although population demographics varied, the populations were found to be similar in sample characteristics. The MDRTC diabetes knowledge test was found to be relable with a Cronbach's alpha = ≥ 0.70 on test items (Fitzgerald et al., 1998). At the same time, the MDRTC diabetes knowledge tool is unable to identify specific components of knowledge and self-care due to its generality (Redman, 2003).

The Arthritis Community Research and Evaluation Unit (ACREU) Rheumatoid Arthritis Knowledge Inventory involves 31 statements that are ranked from strongly agree (one) to strongly disagree (five) (Lineker, Bradley, Hughes, & Bell, 1997; Redman, 2003). The ACREU knowledge tool inventories knowledge in seven areas identified as learning issues by members of a focus group of individuals with rheumatoid arthritis (Lineker, Bradley, Hughes, & Bell, 1997). After the tool was constructed, it was tested for reliablity and validity in a population of 252 patients with rheumatoid athritis in community-based rehabilitation programs or ambulatory or clinical healthcare settings (Lineker, Bradley, Hughes, & Bell, 1997; Redman, 2003). More knowledge is indicated through higher scores, and the highest possible score is 31 (Redman, 2003). In populations of persons with rheumatoid arthritis, the instrument was found to have acceptable internal consistency with a Cronbach's α of 0.76 and a test-retest reliability of 0.92 over 6.7 days (Lineker, Bradley, Hughes, & Bell, 1997). A review of the literature revealed that three studies have been conducted using the ACREU tool (Lineker, Bradley, Hughes, & Bell, 1997; Lineker, Bell, Wilkins, & Bradley, 2001; Bell, Lineker, Wilkins, Goldsmith, & Bradley, 1998).

The Asthma General Knowledge Questionnaire for Adults (AGKQA) is used to evaluate an adult's knowledge of asthma concepts taught in an educational program. The tool was developed by Allen, Jones, and Oldenburg (Allen & Jones, 1998). According to the SMOG readability formula, AGKQA is written at a fifth grade to sixth grade level (Allen & Jones, 1998). The instrument consists of 31 true or false questions; answers may be true, false, or not sure. Not sure answers are used to prevent guessing the correct answer. Only correct true or false answers are given points; not sure and wrong answers are not allotted any points. The total number of correct answers serves as the total score; hence, scores range from 0 to 31. Questions are separated into five content areas, but no subscales are contained in the instrument. The AGKQA was administered to five volunteers to obtain an estimate for time needed to complete the instrument. Completion of the tool takes approximately five to eight minutes. The AGKQA has an internal consistency of 0.56 at baseline (preinstruction) and 0.80 immediately postinstruction (Redman, 2003). A review of the literature revealed the AGKQA has been used in two studies.

The Cardiac Knowledge Questionnaire (CKQ) has 30 true or false questions in the main body (Basic Cardiac Knowledge Scale [BCKS]) with an additional 15 lifestyle questions (Cardiac Lifestyle Knowledge Scale [CLKS]) and 10 misconception questions (Cardiac Misconceptions Scale [CMS]) for a total of 55 items in the measure (Lidell & Fridlund, 1996; Maeland & Havik, 1987). The BCKS and the CLKS together form the Total Cardiac Knowledge Scale (TCKS) while the CMS is separate (Redman, 2003). Content validity for the TCKS was obtained by patients and healthcare professionals, but the 10 CMS questions have not received any measure of validity (Redman, 2003). In a 1987 study, the CKQ tool's internal consistency was determined as BCKS = 0.84, CLKS = 0.69, and CMS = 0.74 (Redman, 2003). A population of 383 post–myocardial infarct patients were used in the original CKQ tool study (Maeland & Havik, 1987). Subjects who did poorly on the misconception questions were found to have decreased expections of regaining preinsult independence and had an increased liklihood of readmission for chest pain not related to cardiac insult (Maeland & Havik, 1987, 1988, 1989). For a period of time, patient education appeared to decrease misconceptions; without educational reinforcement the false impressions returned (Maeland & Havik, 1987, 1988). A literature review found that nine studies have used the CKQ tool to obtain further empirical data.

INCREASED INTEREST IN EVALUATION

Redman (2003) acknowledges that since the publication of the first edition of her book, *Measurement Tools in Patient Education,* which contained 52 instruments, the number of instruments in patient education has almost doubled. She credits this profileration of new measurement tools to the movement of healthcare toward evidence-based practice. One outgrowth of this movement is enhanced interest in patient education or health literacy.

The use of formal assessments and evaluation tools for patient understanding about various phenomena are not standard practices in healthcare (Falvo, 2004; Redman, 2003). Reluctance to use evaluative tools may be attributed to the time commitment of the provider who would be responsible for teaching, administering, and interpreting the results of the intervention (Redman, 2003). In addition, little information about the teacher and the learner, learning conditions, number of teaching or training interactions, amount of time involved in teaching, and testing is included in the publications of the instrument and measurement tool studies. This observation is a common finding across the literature that addresses health literacy in acute and community-based settings. In the future, in order for health literacy to be effective among a diverse patient population, sensitive attention must be given to the development of measures and instruments that are clinically relevant, culturally competent, scientifically robust, and easy to administer, score, and interpret.

PERCEPTION IN EVALUATION

Beyond content intake lies the receiver's comfort with the information and his self-perceived level of mastery. In healthcare, a glimpse into the patient's perception of his understanding of information offers the provider an opportunity to determine where the patient thinks his own knowledge exists on some continuum. Insight into personal perceptions can help the healthcare provider determine what the patient has mastered as well as the areas of deficit. Based on this data, the healthcare provider can develop an intervention that is specific, targeted, and culturally relevant for the patient. Insight into a patient's perception of his ability can help the provider establish a safe environment through appropriate and timely resource utilization. In addition, a provider can note the patient's overall understanding of, and comfort level with, the disease and the prescribed health promotion activities.

The Wong-Baker Pain Scale is a visual tool that provides a medium for patients to communicate their perceived level of pain to healthcare providers and other interested parties. The scale was developed to move beyond the healthcare provider's utilization of observation and personal opinion as an assessment of patients' pain levels. It was specifically thought to be helpful when providing services to pediatric patients, who often have a limited ability to articulate details about their pain and its myriad manifestations. The scale uses six faces that range from a smiling happy face at level 0 to a crying face at level 6 (Wong & Baker, 1988). In practice, the Wong-Baker Pain Scale is a commonly used tool that serves as a standard method for pain assessment across many population groups. The Wong-Baker tool offers a proven, reliable patient perception tool to communicate patients' pain intensity (Kim & Buschmann, 2006; Jansen, 2008; Stubby, 1998). Qualities of the Wong-Baker Pain Scale such as convienience and portability are inviting for clinicians in practice.

The same simple utility of the Wong-Baker scale, if translated into a tool for patient communication of personal perception in understanding and ability, could revolutionize patient education efforts. An understanding of patients' perceptions of their own knowledge and the extent to which they feel able to act could help to improve resource utilization, which has national and global implications. When patient and provider accurately communicate and respect each other, results could include more informed decisions by the patient and the provider, a lower cost of care, and improved mortality and morbidity rates in local and global populations. To this end, the Understanding Personal Perception (UPP) scale has been developed.

UNDERSTANDING PERSONAL PERCEPTION (UPP) SCALE

The Understanding Personal Perception (UPP) Scale was created to offer an alternative method of communicating with patients regarding their level or depth of understanding about particular phenomena related to their health status. It shares the visual feature of a Likert scale measurement that is evident in the Wong-Baker scale (Wong & Baker, 1988). The tool was designed using the sun to represent clarity and clearness, and clouds to represent fuzziness of information and/or confusion about the topic being discussed. Figure 11-1 displays the UPP scale. The sun portrays in-depth understanding of information related to the health condition, while the clouds represent questions and lack of clarity. The sun and cloud images are fashioned in a stair-step manner that is symbolic of upward progression, indicating personal understanding and a sense of self-efficacy. Each step is a numbered point on the five-point Likert scale.

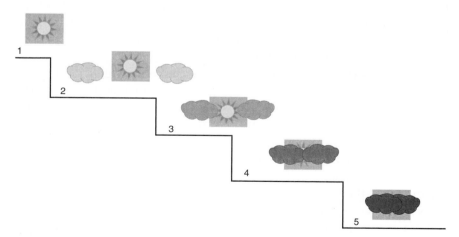

Figure 11-1. The Understanding Personal Perception (UPP) Scale. The sun is representative of clarity of information. The clouds represent confusion, questions, and doubt about the information.

The top level of the scale, level 1, has an image of the sun with no clouds; the correlation is that patients have a comfortable understanding of, or significant clarity about, the content that was introduced in the teaching intervention. In the downward movements, the steps on the scale have cloud images that are intended to indicate a lack of clarify or the incapacity to "understand or see clearly." Notice that the clouds darken and move toward each other, concealing the sun and limiting clarity or the capacity to "see clearly," as the numbers on the scale move downward toward level 5. Ambiguity, the lack of self-efficacy, and limited understanding of the phenomena would be the interpretation of the patient's level of health literacy if level 5 is indicated. On the other hand, the sun, with its entire array of light, suggests that patients' health literacy is high, that self-efficacy is evident, and that self-care could be safely implemented.

As seen in Figure 11-1, clouds are used to represent some level of confusion, lack of understanding, questions, or lack of clarity. The darker the clouds are, the greater the confusion and lack of clarity. Another factor associated with the clouds is the need for resources. The closer and darker the clouds are and the less the sun is seen, the greater the need for assistance through resources. At level 1, complete sun and no clouds requires no resources; the patient is completely independent with the information. Resource requirement increases with movement down toward level 5. At the bottom of the scale complete dependence on healthcare resources is required. Knowing where patients see themselves in their understanding and their ability to act provides insight for the healthcare provider that can be used to safely transition the patient toward an independent state of self-care.

The UPP tool strives to measure the two common themes consistently identified in health literacy: the patient's understanding and the patient's ability to act. The tool uses two questions that the provider asks, and the patient is instructed to point to their answer on the UPP scale. The first question posed to the patient is, "How clear is your present understanding of this information (previously reviewed with or provided to you)?" The patient's answer lets providers know if they can build on present understanding or if they need to clear up any misunderstanding by focusing on areas where there is lack of clarity. The second question is, "How comfortable are you with your understanding and ability to act on or carry out this information?" It is expected that a lack of understanding may influence patients' perceptions of their ability to act. Surprisingly, action is not always contingent on understanding, but action without understanding can pose safety risks. Lack of understanding can serve as a barrier to successful problem solving if any of the patient's circumstances change.

Case Study

Consider Haddie, the retired cafeteria worker who was being trained by her healthcare providers in Chapter 9. As the healthcare providers train Haddie, they use the UPP tool to capture Haddie's perception of her understanding as well as her comfort with carrying out the new behavior. The nurse walks Haddie through the instruction, has her weigh herself, then reviews the parameters of weight gain that should trigger the need for Haddie to call her provider. At that point, the nurse stops to ask Haddie to use the UPP tool to identify where she feels she is in her understanding. While holding up the tool, the nurse asks Haddie, "How clear is your present understanding of this information I reviewed with you?" Haddie reveals that she's at a level 3 in understanding how to weigh herself and a level 4 regarding when to call. The nurse then asks, "How comfortable are you with your understanding and ability to do this by yourself?" Haddie gives herself a 4 in weighing and a 5 in calling.

By using the UPP tool, the healthcare provider gained insight into Haddie's perception of her understanding and ability to act upon the new information. This information can help the healthcare provider become aware of the resources the patient needs to assist her in carrying out the activity.

The nurse, in collaboration with the patient, decides to follow up with Haddie in a call to review information and walk Haddie through each step of the weigh and call process. The next day the nurse calls at the established time. Haddie is able to successfully weigh herself and correctly determines that she is not in the parameters that would trigger a phone call to report weight-gain. The nurse then asks Haddie to rescale herself using the UPP tool. Haddie picks up the copy of the UPP tool the nurse gave her. On reevaluation, Haddie scales her understanding at 2 and her ability to act at 2. The nurse makes sure Haddie has her contact number and tells Haddie that she will call her next week to how things are going. The following week's call reveals that Haddie has been successful in her weight monitoring.

BEYOND THE BEDSIDE

One of the challenges associated with health literacy is how best to communicate with patients and connect with their personal view within the context of improving health. The UPP Scale provides unique insight into where patients envision their understanding and their ability to act upon their understanding. Although the conception of the UPP scale originated in healthcare as a tool to be used between the patient and the provider, its use is not limited to the healthcare setting. Portability and ease of use make the tool attractive. The UPP tool can be used with any information, in any setting, and for any person. The tool's design allows it to be administered in minimal time, ideally less than a minute. From the academic classroom to the hospital room, anywhere clear communication and understanding is needed the tool can be used. Within the healthcare setting, patient satisfaction, effectiveness of patient teaching, and many unseen factors may become apparent with insight into patient perception.

There is abundant evidence to support the benefits that patient education brings to health outcomes (Falvo, 2004; Osborne, 2005; Redman, 2004). Redman (2003) mentions that patient education is routinely practiced in the healthcare setting without a common methodology or approach, and that healthcare system changes will necessitate system-wide recognition of a universal methodical approach to patient education. In the Centers for Medicare and Medicaide Services (CMS) care transitions pilot, the UPP scale helped CPEs and Patient Specialist coaches identify appropriate follow-up time frames. Recognizing where patients saw themselves in knowledge and ability aided in transitioning patients into self-care safely. The UPP scale provided valuable insight that helped in care coordination so healthcare providers could provide timely and appropriate intervention and avoid unnecessary readmissions. Insight into patients' perceived gains in their understanding of health information can assist providers in meeting patients' resource needs and improve patient outcomes.

SUMMARY

- As healthcare becomes more patient oriented, providers will have to treat each patient as an individual. The aspiration of a new patient-oriented community of care can only become reality by addressing each patient's health literacy needs.

- The medagogy framework offers a pathway for educating individuals and can be beneficial in management of chronic illness. Treatment and management of chronic illness translates financially into more than 1 trillion dollars of the annual federal healthcare budget.

- Patient education should include evaluative techniques to assess patient understanding. Historically, standard knowledge measurement that is traditional to academic settings has not been used in healthcare.

- Universally, health literacy definitions acknowledge patients' needs to understand and utilize health information to which they have been exposed. Feldman and McPhee (2008) acknowledge that comprehension and understanding are abstract; therefore, direct measurement is often challenging.

- In healthcare, the patient's perception of his personal understanding of information offers the provider an opportunity to determine where the patient thinks his knowledge exists on some continuum. Insight into personal perceptions can help the healthcare provider determine what the patient has mastered as well as the areas of deficits. Based on this data, the healthcare provider can develop an intervention that is specific, targeted, and culturally relevant for the patient.

- The Wong-Baker Pain Scale offers a proven and reliable patient perception tool to communicate patients' pain intensity.

- The simple utility of the Wong-Baker scale, translated into a tool for patient communication of personal perception, could revolutionize patient education efforts.

- The Understanding Personal Perception (UPP) scale offers an alternative method of communicating with patients regarding their level or depth of understanding about particular phenomena related to their health status. It shares the visual feature with a Likert scale measurement that is evident in the Wong-Baker scale.

- The UPP tool was designed using a sun and clouds to represent clarity and clearness, or fuzziness and confusion of information and depth of understanding about the topic being discussed.

- The sun and cloud images are fashioned in a stair-step manner that is symbolic of upward progression, indicating personal understanding and a sense of self-efficacy. Each step is a numbered point on the five-point Likert scale.

- The UPP tool strives to measure the two common themes consistently identified in health literacy: understanding and ability to act.

- The tool uses two questions that the provider asks the patient:
  1. "How clear is your present understanding of this information (previously reviewed with or provided to you)?" This lets providers know if they can build on present understanding or if they need to clear up any misunderstanding by focusing on areas where there is lack of clarity.
  2. "How comfortable are you with your understanding and ability to act on or carry out this information?" It is expected that a lack of understanding may influence the patients' perceptions of their ability to act. Surprisingly, action is not always contingent on understanding, but action without understanding can pose safety risks.
- One of the challenges associated with health literacy is how best to communicate with patients and connect with their personal view within the context of improving health.
- The UPP tool provides unique insight into where patients envision their understanding and ability. Although the conception of the UPP tool originated in healthcare as a tool to be used between the patient and the provider, its use is not limited to the healthcare setting. Portability and ease of use make the tool attractive anywhere clear communication and understanding is needed.
- In the Centers for Medicare and Medicaide Services (CMS) care transitions pilot, the UPP scale aided in transitioning patients into self-care safely and helped in care coordination so healthcare providers intervened in a timely and appropriate way to avoid unnecessary readmissions.

SECTION IV SUMMARY

Patient education empowers the patient with health autonomy through personal health knowledge. The process of patients arriving at their health-care decisions, according to medagogy, is intimately connected to patient health knowledge, individualism, and the weight of external and internal influences. The patient education model PITS offers a pathway for health-care providers to use when educating patients. Medagogy offers an over-arching framework for patient education conceptual structures. Medagogy offers insight into an unprecented theoretical view of patient internalization of information as the patient maneuvers through influences and generates personal healthcare decisions.

Whereas health literacy aims to identify patient deficits in the knowledge of health, medagogy focuses on the method by which patient individualism is central to patient understanding in the education process, thus promoting patient literacy. Medagogy focuses on providers meeting patients at the patients' level of health knowledge, transitioning the inter-action to patient-centered information exchange. The UPP scale allows the healthcare provider to gain insight into patients' perceptions and comfort with their ability to act upon information. Tools found in the research literature are long, cumbersome, not well utilized in the healthcare setting, and are disease rather than patient focused.

The simplicity of the Wong-Baker Pain Scale along with its ability to capture patients' perception provided the impetus for the UPP scale. The UPP scale uses pictures of clouds and the sun to signify clarity of under-standing.

While an abundance of data regarding health literacy and patient education can be found in the literature, standard universal strategic patient education delivery remains inconsistent at the point of service in daily practice. Illumination of the profundity of this healthcare problem should inspire the need for immediate action to progress patient knowledge as the result of patient-centered education via established patient-provider part-nership. Peer interpretation is encouraged and welcomed as the role of the patient educator evolves through evidence-based practice. No two patients are exactly the same, and no two patient educational sessions should be identical.

AUTHOR'S FINAL THOUGHTS

We can no longer just treat; we must teach and reach every patient. Through understanding our patients as individuals, we can give them a sense of personal priority and health direction. Prescriptive precedence is an exercise in futility. Only through shared knowledge and partnership in healthcare decision making can optimal healthcare outcomes be attained. PITS allows patients to see "behind the curtain" by exposing them to expert knowledge that drives healthcare decisions. The informational seasons, hierarchy of patient education, medagogy conceptual framework, and UPP scale all serve to help the provider center information around the patient rather than around the elusive concept of health.

The UPP Tool Pilot

Annette Knobloch, DNS, RN, MPH, CNE, CPST
Associate Professor, Our Lady of the Lake College

Preliminary psychometric properties of an adapted version of Stewart's Understanding Personal Perception (UPP) scale were tested with a small sample ($N = 15$) of nurse educators in conjunction with Knobloch's (2010, March 15) continuing education session, "You and the Registry of Nursing Research Database, Virginia Henderson International Nursing Library, Sigma Theta Tau International." The study was approved by the Our Lady of the Lake College Institutional Review Board. Participants received a study packet consisting of pretest and posttest study forms, and the traditional Continuing Education Participant Evaluation form (CEPE, Our Lady of the Lake Health Career Institute). The forms in each packet were pre-coded with matching study numbers, which ensured anonymity while allowing the linkage of the three study forms to responders. Participation was optional, and completion of the forms constituted consent.

The pretest and posttest study forms consisted of the pictorial UPP rating scale placed horizontally below each of the six session objectives, such that there were six rows, each with a session objective and the UPP images. Stewart's UPP numeric ratings ranged from 1 to 5, with 1 representing the brightest sunshine image, and 6 representing the darkest clouds. Therefore lower scores indicated higher perceived understanding. The CEPE contained three sections:

- A block for rating the *achievement* of the same six session objectives, with a Likert scale worded Excellent, Good, Fair, Poor, n/a. Responses were coded 1, 2, 3, 4, respectively, and lower ratings indicated higher ratings. There were no participants who chose "n/a" (not applicable) responses.

- A block with the Likert scale ratings for the instructor's knowledge of content, presentation skills, and organization of content.
- A block with five overall program objectives related to the extend to which the session met expectations, the quality of the session and handouts, and the impact of the session on the participant. Three relevant sub-items from the impact-related CEPE statement were treated as separate items in various analyses in this study: (a) increase your knowledge? (b) change a skill or attitude? and (c) change your practice performance?

The three study forms had high internal consistency values. Reliability and factor analyses (Table A-1) were performed for the pretest form the posttest form, and the CEPE form despite the small sample size for several reasons. First, conducting these analyses necessitated the setting up of data entry and data processing for potential use in future studies with larger samples and to provide results for this particular study. Second, there were no psychometric data available for the CEPE, and these analyses provided information for relevant sections of the CEPE for this study. Data from the six objective-related items in the first block and the three components of impact-related statement were compiled and utilized for analyses in this study. Thus, CEPE items that were conceptually unrelated to the UPP were excluded, and the findings herein reported for the CEPE apply to the portions of the CEPE used in various study analyses. Despite the small sample size, principal component factor analysis, with varimax rotation, of the posttest UPP data supported construct validity: Kaiser-Meyer-Olkin (KMO) Measure of Sampling Adequacy (MSA) values, overall and per objective, were greater than .5, as were the communalities for each objective. A single factor emerged with loadings ranging from .79 to .97.

A paired samples t-test revealed significantly higher ratings on the posttest, compared to the pretest, for each objective, and for the set of objectives $t(14)$ ranged from 3.3 to 5.3, p ranged from < .001 to .005, and no confidence intervals for the mean difference contained zero. The p values were all less than .007, and thus were still significant at the overall .05 level after the Bonferroni adjustment for multiple comparisons. Higher posttest ratings provided additional support for construct validity for use of the UPP as a rating scale because it was expected that the participants' ratings for the session objectives would be higher after the session than before the session. The pretest and posttest study forms, using UPP as a rating scale in conjunction with the stated objectives, were able to detect differences in perceived understanding before and after the continuing education session.

Table A-1 Summary of Psychometric Properties for Forms in this Study, $N = 15$

Form	Items	Cronbach's Alpha	Factor Analysis					
			Factors	Range of Item Loadings on Factor	Variance Explained	KMO	Range of MSA Values	Range of Communalities
Pretest	6	.98	One	.89 to .98	90.4%	*	*	.80 to .96
Posttest	6	.95	One	0.79 to 0.97	82.6%	.85	.78 to .97	.62 to .94
CEPE Block 1	6	.98	One	0.91 to 0.97	91.5%	*	.77 to .91	.52 to .96
CEPE Block 1 and Impact items	9	.91	Two	.89 to .99 (objective items). .81 to .91 (impact items)	88.9%	*	*	.84 to .97

*Undeterminable, probably due to very small sample size.
KMO (Kaiser-Meyer-Olkin) and MSA (measure of sampling adequacy) refer, respectively, to overall and individual item indices that aid in determining whether factor analysis is advisable.

The Pearson correlations between the UPP and CEPE ratings were not significant, ranging from -0.08 to 0.35, with p values ranging from .19 to .76. These nonsignificant correlations supported discriminate validity, because the UPP measured *perception* of understanding related to the session objectives, but the CEPE measured *achievement*.

In summary, these findings demonstrate the effectiveness of the UPP rating scale for this study and provide support for additional testing of the tool with adequate sample sizes, various populations, and various research questions.

Laurie's Story from the Care Transitions' Pilot

Laurie Robinson, RN, CPE, CPUR, Director of Quality, eQHealth Solutions QIO

I arrived at 9 AM for a two-and-a-half-day training on patient education. As a registered nurse with 25 years of experience, I thought this would be a great opportunity to brush up on my skills in this area. I had taken on a new project as part of the work I was doing at eQHealth Solutions. The project was designed to address transitions of patients after discharge from the hospital in an effort to reduce avoidable readmission. One of the interventions that I had implemented in the community was transition coaching. I remember thinking that the patient education class might help me in this project, and if not, at least I would have all the Continuing Education Units I needed to renew my license.

Two hours into the training, I felt myself tightening up. "We do this already," I thought. With all that I had on my plate, every moment was precious, and I hoped that sitting through this Certified Patient Education course would be a valuable investment. I hoped I wasn't wasting my time. On day two of training I challenged medagogy and the PITS model, thinking, "It can't be this simple. Surely we are already covering this information in patient education." Unbeknownst to me, my assumptions about patient education were not in touch with what was happening at the bedside. I completed the course, passed the exam, and was officially a Certified Patient Educator (CPE). I committed myself to putting this model to the test.

The transition coaching intervention is designed to provide support to patients in the vulnerable 30–45 day period after discharge. The CPE or Patient Specialist transitions coach meets with patients while they are in the hospital and follows up via telephone after discharge. The interactions focus on the discharge plan of care, medication reconciliation, a follow-up appointment with the patient's physician, a patient personal health record, warning signs, and a patient-centered goal. I was mentoring a new coach as we were kicking off the intervention in an acute care hospital. This is where I realized that, as providers, we had veered off the path regarding patient education.

My new coach and I met with our first patient, Jane Doe, who was referred to our program with a diagnosis of congestive heart failure (CHF). The treatment team described her as a "frequent flyer" since she was regularly hospitalized at least four times a year. "If she would just stop drinking those Diet Cokes and eating animal crackers, she would not need to keep coming to the hospital," was uttered in the report that I received from the nurse. I entered the room to find a 54-year-old female who was admitted with CHF, but who also was suffering from chronic obstructive pulmonary disease (COPD), hypertension, and insulin-dependent diabetes. Her husband had died two years earlier while in hospice with end-stage COPD. She was raising her two grandchildren, who were ages 9 and 12, because, as she put it, "My daughter loves crack more than she loves her children." She also had a 26-year-old daughter living with her who was disabled from a closed head injury. As I listened to her, I thought to myself, "And we think it's animal crackers and Diet Coke?"

I started to work with Jane using the principles I had learned in my CPE training. I don't know whether my senses were heightened to the problem since acquiring my new title of CPE or if, like everyone else, I had become somewhat desensitized to patient educational needs. Either way, I quickly noticed that something was missing. I realized when I was talking with the patient about her warning signs that something wasn't clicking. So I asked the patient whether she could tell me what was wrong with her heart pump. "There's nothing wrong with my heart pump," she replied. So I asked in a different way. Same answer. I was astonished. How could someone with stage IV heart failure not know what was wrong with her heart pump? Granted, Jane Doe was a high school graduate of low socioeconomic status, but certainly with all the clinicians with whom she had interacted over the many years, someone must have provided her with information about her disease so that she would know what was wrong with her heart's ability to work as a pump. I decided this would be the perfect patient with whom to put the medagogy methodology, specifically the PITS model, to the test.

I started to teach using my fist as the model of the heart—not a great deal of anatomic information, but just enough to cover basic pathophysiology. Jane Doe did not know that when you have CHF, your heart pump will not get better. Where did we miss the boat? Every day I refreshed her on the information I had covered and began to build on it like the PITS model recommends. From the very first learning interaction, I noticed that Jane's body language began to change as she became empowered with information. She made eye contact, she sat up taller, she asked questions, she did exactly what we want in coaching and in healthcare: she engaged with me.

As I taught and quizzed her and she succeeded, she became more confident. We covered pathophysiology, indications, treatment, and specifics of diagnosis that were unique to her. Jane remarked, "Only my right hand and leg swell when I am starting to get into trouble with my heart." Her ability to identify her individual body's response to her diagnosis indicated to me that we were moving in the right direction. I returned on a Monday to visit Jane only to find her in a great deal of distress. She was having difficulty breathing; she was leaning over the bedside table and appeared to be exhausted. They had administered oxygen, which she reported was not helping. When I asked her what she thought the problem was, she replied, "I have gained nine pounds." "Nine pounds," I responded. She told me she had gained nine pounds and she knew the reason. "Why do you think you have gained so much weight in such a short period of time?" I asked. Jane told me that, since they had transferred her to skilled care, that they had not been giving her the water pill that she normally took. I checked the medical record and saw that it was not continued at the time of transfer. I thought to myself, "Would this patient before our teaching sessions have made the connection between the breathing difficulty and the water pill?" I informed the charge nurse of the findings. She assured me she would call the physician and get orders for a diuretic. I went back to Jane and asked her whether she could talk with her doctor about this when he visited and she agreed to do so.

I returned the next day to find Jane not happy about having spent all night in the bathroom. I asked her how her conversation with the doctor had gone. Unfortunately, I learned that the charge nurse had become busy and had not contacted the doctor. When Jane informed the doctor of the medication mishap, he challenged her. She explained the events leading up to our discovery. He checked the medical record and told Jane that she was correct. Most often patients do not challenge the treatment team especially in the hospital setting. Jane felt confident because she was knowledgeable. Jane's new confidence paid off. She was now taking the lead in her care—so much so that she asked the social worker what she could do to stay out of the hospital. She wanted to be at home with her grandchildren. She knew that her heart was not going to return to the way that it was when it was healthy: her heart was diseased and it would stay diseased. The social worker discussed hospice options. Jane agreed to an informational visit and, after meeting with the hospice nurse, decided that hospice was her best option. Since Jane was discharged from our coaching program over a year ago, she has not been admitted to the hospital, is experiencing better symptom management, and has negated avoidable re-hospitalizations.

I was amazed at this patient's relative lack of knowledge regarding her condition. During the implementation of the intervention at the hospital I decided to ask other patients with heart failure to describe the problem with their heart pump. Surely Jane was an exception. Unfortunately, this was not so. After questioning 10 patients, all of whom could not explain what was wrong with their heart, I decided that our coaching model needed to include the medagogy framework and that the PITS model and the Understanding Personal Perspective (UPP) scale needed to be the platform for all patient education efforts.

I don't know how we became so disconnected from patients but it is evident when you look at patient education today. The PITS model affords us a structured delivery that meets patients' needs at any point that we interact with our patients. Components of the medagogy framework, the PITS model, the patient education hierarchy, and the Understanding Personal Perspective (UPP) scale all serve to foster knowledge, understanding, confidence, and behavior change. There are many Jane Does out there who need our help. Healthcare providers need to embrace and believe in the power of the knowledgeable patient.

[REFERENCES]

"Access". (2005). Access program reduces inappropriate admissions. *Hospital Case Management, 13*(5), 69–75.

Ajzen, I., & Fishbein, M. (1980). *Understanding attitudes and predicting social behavior.* Englewood Cliffs, NJ: Prentice-Hall.

Albert, N.M., Buchsbaum, R., & Li, J. (2007). Randonized study on the effect of video education on heart failure healthcare utilization, symptoms, and self-care behaviors. *Patient Education and Counseling, 69*(1), 129–139.

Albon, A. (2008). Reconstructing recall: room for improvement? Amanda Albon describes how psychologists have used knowledge about how memory works to improve the accuracy of eyewitness recall. *Psychology Review, 13*(3), 24–26.

Alexander, R. (2004). Still no pedagogy? Principle, pragmatism, and compliance in primary education. *Cambridge Journal of Education, 34*(1), 7–30.

Allen, R.M., & Jones, M.P. (1998). The validity and reliability for asthma knowledge questionnaire used in the evaluation of a group asthma self-management program for adults with asthma. *Journal of Asthma, 35*(7), 537–545.

American Hospital Association. (1973). *A patient's bill of rights.* Retrieved from http://www.patienttalk.info/AHA-Patient_Bill_of_Rights.htm

American Medical Association Ad Hoc Committee on Health Literacy for the Council on Scientific Affairs, (1999). Health literacy: Report of the council of scientific affairs. *Journal of the American Medical Association, 281*(6), 552–557.

American Nurses Association. (2004). *Nursing: Scope and standards of practice.* Washington, DC: Nursesbooks.org.

Anderson, J.G., Rainey, M.R., & Eysenbach, G. (2004). The impact of cyberhealth on the physician-patient relationship. *Journal of Medical Systems, 27*(1), 67–84.

Anderson, L.W., Krathwohl, D.R., Airsian, P.W., Cruikshank, K.A., Mayer, R.E., Pintrich, P.R.,...Wittrock, M.C. (Eds.). (2001). *A taxonomy for learning, teaching, and assessment: A revision of Bloom's taxonomy of educational objectives.* New York: Longman

Anderson, R.C., & Speiro, R.J. (1977). *Schooling and the acquisition of knowledge.* Hillsdale, NJ: Erlbaum.

Anderson, R.C., Spiro, R.J., & Montague, W.W. (Eds.). (1984). *Schooling and the acquisition of knowledge.* Hillsdale, NJ: Erlbaum.

Anonymous. (2009, September). Matching teaching strategies with adult learning styles maximizes education effectiveness. *Strategies for Nurse Managers, 9*(9), 7–9.

Aristole. (2009). *Metaphysics.* (W.D. Ross, Trans.) U.S.: Classics-Unbound.

Atherton J.S. (2009). Learning and teaching: Misrepresentation, myths and misleading ideas Retrieved from http://www.learningandteaching.info/learning/myths.htm

Ausubel, D.P., Novak, J.D., & Hanesian, H. (1986). Educational psychology: A cognitive view (2nd ed.). New York, NY: Werbel & Peck.

Avillion, A.E. (2009, October). Tailor education to appeal to all adult learning styles. HCPro's Advisor to the ANCC Magnet Recognition Program, *5*(10), 6.

Avillion, A.E. (2009). *Learning styles in nursing education: Integrating teaching strategies into staff development.* Marblehead, MA: HCPro.

Bacon, F. (1893). *The advancement of learning.* (D. Price, Trans.) U.K.: Cassell & Company.

Bailey, R.N. (1995). Community-oriented primary care programs. *Journal of American Optometric Association, 66*(10), 631–633.

Baker, D.W. (2006). The meaning and measure of health literacy. *Journal of General Internal Medicine, 21*(8), 878–883.

Baker, D.W., Gazmararian, J.A., Williams, M.V., Scott, T., Parker, R.M., & Green, D.,...Ren, J. (2002). Functional health literacy and the risk of hospital admission among Medicare managed care enrollees. *American Journal of Public Health, 92*(8), 1278–1283.

Balota, D.A., & Marsh, E.J. (2004). *Cognitive Psychology: Key Readings.* Taylor & Francis. Retrieved from http://lib.myilibrary.com/Browse/open.asp?ID=28915&loc=659

Bandura, A. (1977). *Social Learning Theory.* New York, NY: General Learning Press.

Bandura, A. (1994). Self-efficacy. In V.S. Ramachaudran (Ed.), *Encyclopedia of humanbehavior* (Vol. 4, pp. 71–81). New York, NY: Academic Press. (Reprinted in H. Friedman [Ed.], *Encyclopedia of mental health.* San Diego: Academic Press, 1998).

Bandura, A. (1997). *Self-efficacy: The exercise of control.* New York, NY: W.H. Freeman.

Barlett, E.E. (1986). Historical glimpses of patient education in the United States. *Patient Education and Counseling, 8*(2), 135–149.

Barrett, S.E., & Puryear, J.S. (2006). Health literacy: Improving quality of care in primary care settings. *Journal of Health Care for the poor and underserved, 17*(4), 690–697.

Bash, L. (2005). *Best practices in adult learning*. Bolton, MA: Anker Publishing Co.

Bastable, S.B. (2006). Essentials of Patient Education. Sudbury, MA: Jones and Barlett.

Bauer, P.J., (1996). What do infants recall of their lives? Memory for specific events by one- to two-year-old. *American Psychologist, 51*(1), 29–41.

Baum, M. (2005). *Understanding behaviorism*. Malden, MA: Blackwell Publishing.

Bayliss, E.A., Ellis, J.L., & Steiner, J.F. (2007). Barriers to self-management and quality-of-life outcomes in seniors with multimorbidities. *Annuals of Family Medicine, 5*(5), 395–402.

Becker, M.H. (Ed.). (1974). "The Health Belief Model and Personal Health Behavior." *Health Education Monographs, 2*(4), 324–473.

Becker, M.H., Kaback, M.M, Rosenstock, I.M., & Ruth, M.V. (1975). Some influences on public participation in a genetic screening program. *Journal of Community Health, 1*(1), 3–14

Becker, M.H., Nathanson, C.A., Drachman, R.H., & Kirscht, J.P. (1977). Mothers' health beliefs and children's clinic visits: A prospective study. *Journal of Community Health, 3*(2),125–135.

Behar-Horenstein, L.S., Guin, P., Gamble, K., Hurlock, G., Leclear, E., Philipose, M.,...Weldon, J. (2005). Improving care through patient and family education programes. *Hospital Topics, 83*(1), 21–27.

Beisecker, A.E., & Beisecker, T.D. (1990). Patient information-seeking behaviours when communicating with doctors. *Medical Care, 28*(1), 19–28.

Bell, M.J., Lineker, S.C., Goldsmith, C.H., & Badley, E.M., (1998). A Randomized Controlled Trial to Evaluate the Efficacy of Community Based Physical Therapy in the Treatment of People with Rheumatoid Arthritis. *The Journal of Rheumatology, 25*(2), 231–237.

Bensing, J. (2000). Bridging the gap: The separate worlds of evidence-based medicine and patient-centered medicine. *Patient Education and Counseling, 39*(1), 17–25.

Best, J.T. (2001). Effective teaching for elderly: Back to basics. *Orthopaedic Nursing, 20*(3), 46–52.

Betz, C.L., Ruccione, K., Meeske, K., Smith, K., & Chang, N. (2008). Health literacy: A pediatric nursing concern. *Pediatric Nursing, 34*(3), 231–239.

Beyer, H.S. (2009). The 300-year-old health care solution. *Archives of Internal Medicine, 169*(19), 1818.

Billek-Sawhney, B., & Reicherter, E.A. (2005). Literacy and the older adult: Educational considerations for health professionals. *Topics in Geriatric Rehabilitation, 21*(4), 275–281.

Bishop, G.D. (1991). Understanding the understanding of illness: Lay disease representations. In J.A. Skelton, & R.T. Croyle (Eds.), *Mental Representation in Health and Illness* (pp. 32–60). New York: Springer.

Bishop, V. (2009). Leaders of the Future. *Nursing Standards, 24*(10), 62–63.

Bloom, B. (1956). *Taxonomy of educational objectives: The classification of educational goals.* New York, NY: Longman Publishing Group.

Boberg, E.W., Gustafson, D.H., Hawkins, R.P., Offord, K.P., Koch, C., & Wen, K.Y.,...Salner, A. (2003). Assessing the unmet information, support and care delivery needs of men with prostate cancer. *Patient Education and Counseling, 49*(3), 233–242.

Bodenheimer, T., & Fernandez, A. (2005). High and rising health care costs: Can costs be controlled while preserving quality? Part 4. *Annals of Internal Medicine, 143*(1), 26–31.

Bolman, C., Brug, J., Bar, J., & Van de Borne, B. (2005). Long-term efficacy of a checklist to improve patient education in cardiology. *Patient Education and Counseling, 56*(2), 240–248.

Boothman, N. (2002). *How to connect in business in 90 seconds or less.* New York, NY: Workman Publishing Company, Inc.

Boreham, P., & Gibson, D. (1978). The informative process in private medical consultations: A preliminary investigation. *Social Science and Medicine, 12*(5), 409–416.

Boren, S.A., Wakefield, B.J., Gunlock, T.L., & Wafefield, D.S. (2009). Heart failure self-management education: a systematic review of the evidence. [Miscellaneous Article]. *International Journal of Evidence-Based Healthcare, 7*(3), 159–168.

Boswell, C., Cannon, S., Aung, K., & Eldridge, J. (2004). An application of health literacy research. *Applied Nursing Research, 17*(1), 61–64.

Bower, G.H., & Hilgard, E.R., (1981). *Theories of learning* (5th ed.). Englewood Cliffs, NJ: Prentice Hall.

Boyd, M.D., Gleit, C.J., Graham, B.A., & Whitman, N.L. (1998). *Health teaching in nursing practice: A professional model* (3rd ed.). Stamford, CT: Appleton & Lange.

Boyde, M., Tuckett, A., Peters, R., Thompson, D., Turner, C., & Stewart, S. (2009). Learning for heart failure patients (The L-HF study). *The Journal of Clinical Nursing, 18*(14), 2030.

Breslow, L. (1999). From disease prevention to health promote. *Journal of the American Medical Association, 281*(11), 1030–1033.

Brey, R.A., Clark, S.E., & Wantz, M.S. (2007). Enhancing health literacy through accessing health information, products, and services: An exercise for children and adolescents. *Journal of School Health, 77*(9), 640–644.

Brey, R.A., Clark, S.E., & Wantz, M.S. (2008). This is your future: A case study approach to foster health literacy. *Journal of School Health, 78*(6), 351–355.

Brodenheimer, T., Lorig, K., Holman, H., & Grumbach, K. (2002). Patient self-management of chronic disease in primary care. *The Journal of the American Medical Association, 288*(19), 2469–2475.

Brookfield, S.D. (2006). *The skillful teacher: On technique, trust, and responsiveness in the classroom* (2nd ed.). San Francisco, CA: Jossey-Bass.

Brown, A.L., (1978). Knowing when, where and how to remember: A problem of metacognition. In R. Glaser (Ed.), *Advances in instructional psychology*. Hillsdale, NJ: Erlbaum.

Brown, S.L., Teufel, J.A., & Birch, D.A. (2007). Early adolescents perceptions of health literacy. *Journal of School Health, 77*(1), 7–15.

Brunetti, L. & Hermes-DeSantis, E. (2010). The internet as a drug information resource. *US Pharmacist, 35*(1). Retrieved December 11, 2011 from http://prod.uspharmacist.com/content/c/19130/

Brunner, J., (1990). *Acts of meaning*. Cambridge, MA: Harvard University Press.

Bucy, P.C., (1981). Ancora impero –I continue to learn. *Neurologia Medico-chirurgica, 21*(7):629–34

Bull, F.C., Kreuter, M.W., & Scharff, D.P. (1999). Effects of tailored, personalized and general health messages on physical activity. *Patient Education and Counseling, 36*(2), 181–192.

Burnham, E., & Peterson, E.B. (2005). Health information literacy: A library case study. *Library Trends, 53*(3), 422–433.

Bybee, R. (Ed.). (1966). *National Standards and the Science Curriculum: Challenges, Opportunities, and Recommendations*. Dubuque, Iowa: Kendall-Hunt.

Cagle, J.G., & Kovacs, P.J. (2009). Education: A complex and empowering social work intervention at end of life. *Health & Social Work, 34*(1), 17–27.

California State University, Northridge (2008). *What is a CHES?*. Retrieved from MPH Program: http://www.csun.edu/~hchsc006/id42.htm

Calvin, W.H. (1995). *How Brains Think: Evolving Intelligence, Then and Now*. New York, NY: Basic Books.

Campbell, E.M., Redman, S., Moffitt, P.S., & Sanson-Fisher, R.W. (1996). The relative effectiveness of educational and behavioral instruction programs for patients with N1DDM: A randomized trial. *The Diabetes Educator, 22*, 379–386.

Campbell, R.J. (2008). Meeting seniors' information needs: Using computer technology. *Home Health Care Management and Practice, 4*, 328–335.

Campbell, S.M., Roland, M.O., Middleton, E., & Reeves, D. (2005). Improvements in quality of clinical care in English general practice 1998–2003: Longitudinal observational study. *BMJ, 331*, 1121. doi:10.1136/bmj.38632.611123

Canadian Public Health Association, Report of Expert panel (2008) A vision for a health literate Canada. Author. Retrieved December 6, 2011, from http://www.cpha.ca/uploads/portals/h-l/report_e.pdf

Cannick, G.F., Horowitz, A.M., Garr, D.R., Reed, S.G., Neville, B.W., Day, T.A., & ... Lackland, D.T. (2007). Oral cancer prevention and early detection: Using the PRECEDE-PROCEED framework to guide the training of health professional students. *Journal Of Cancer Education, 22*(4), 250–253.

Carter, N.J., & Wallace, R.L. (2007). Collaborating with public libraries, public health departments, and rural hospitals to provide consumer health information services. *Journal of Consumer Health on the Internet, 11*(4), 1–14.

Center for Health Strategies, Inc. (2005). *What is health literacy?* [Fact sheet]. Retrieved from http://www.chcs.org/usr_doc/Health_Literacy_Fact_Sheets.pdf

Centers for Disease Control (2007). *Healthy People 2010.* Retrieved from Centers for Disease Control: http://www.cdc.gov/nchs/about/otheract/hpdata2010/abouthp.htm

Chang, B.L., Bakken, S., Brown, S.S., Houston, T.K., Kreps, G.L., Kukafka, R.,... Stavri, P.Z. (2004). Bridging the digital divide: Reaching vulnerable populations. *Journal of the American Medical Informatics Association, 11*(6), 448–457.

Chang, M., & Kelly, A.E. (2007). Patient education: Addressing cultural diversity and health literacy issues. *Urologic Nursing, 27*(5), 411–417.

Chase, W.G., & Simon, H.A. (1973). Perception in chess. *Cognitive Psychology, 4,* 55–81.

Chomsky, N. (1959). Review of Skinner's *verbal behavior. Language, 35,* 26–58

Clark, N.M., & Gong, M. (2000). Management of chroinc diseases by practitioners and patients: Are we teaching the wrong things? *BMJ, 320,* 572–575.

Clark, N.M., Gong, M., Schork, M.A., Evans, D., Roloff, D., Hurwitz, M.,... Mellins, R.B.(1997). Impact education for physicians on patient outcomes. *Pediatrics, 101*(5), 831–836.

Clark, P.A., Drain, M., & Malone, M.P. (2003). Addressing patients' emotional and spiritual needs. *Joint Commission Journal on Quality and Safety, 29*(12), 659–670.

Close, A. (1988). Patient education: A literature review. *Journal of Advanced Nursing, 13*(2), 203–213.

CMS (2011) HCACPS: Patients perspectives of care survey. Retrieved from CMS. gov on December 10, 2011 from: https://www.cms.gov/HospitalQualityInits/30_HospitalHCAHPS.asp

Coates, H. (2007), Integrating patient-centered care and evidence-based practices: What is the prognosis for healthcare? (Unpublished research paper) Indiana University, Indianapolis. Retrieved December 11,2011 from: http://home.com-cast.net/~h.coates/S653-PCC+EBP.pdf

Cognitivism. (2004). In *Encyclopedia of Applied Psychology.* Retrieved from http://www.credoreference.com/entry/estappliedpsyc/cognitivism

Collins, A.S., Gullette, D., & Schnepf, M. (2005). Break through language barriers. *Nurse Practitioners: The 2005 sourcebook for advanced practice nurses, 30*(suppl 1), 19–20.

Committee on Health Literacy. (2004, April 8). *Health Literacy: A prescription to end confusion* (The Institute of Medicine of the National Academies). Washington DC: The National Academies Press.

Committee on Understanding and Eliminating Racial and Ethnic Disparities in Health Care. (2003). *Unequal Treatment: Confronting Racial and Ethnic Disparities in Health Care.* (B.D. Smedley, A. Stith, & A. Nelson, Eds.) Washington DC: the National Academies Press.

Conti, G., & Welborn, R. (1986). Teaching learning styles and the adult learner. *Lifelong Learning, 9*(8), 20–24.

Cooper, H., Booth, K., Fear, S., & Gill, G. (2001). Chronic disease patient education: Lessons from meta-analyses. *Patient Education and Counseling, 44*(2), 107–117.

Costa, M.L., Rensburg, L.V., & Rushton, N., (2007). Does teaching style matter? A randomised trial of group discussion versus lectures in orthopaedic undergraduate teaching. *Medical Education, 41*(2), 214–217. doi: 10.1111/j.1365–2929.2007.02700.x

Cowan, N. (2001). The magical number of 4 in short-term memory: A reconsideration of mental storage capacity. *Behavioral and Brain Sciences, 24*(1), 87–114.

Create a standard for communication despite patient's level of health literacy. (2008). *Patient Education Management, 15*(4), 37–38.

Cromie, W.J. (2006, July 10). *The longer you live the long you can expect to live.* Retrieved from Harvard University Gazette, Retrieved December 11, 2011: http://www.news.harvard.edu/gazette/2006/07.20/10-deathquiz.html

Curry, L.C., Walker, C., Hogstel, M.O., & Burns, P. (2005). Teaching older adults to self-manage medications: Preventing adverse drug reactions. *Journal of Gerontological Nursing, 31*(4), 32–42.

Curtis, J.R., Patrick, D.L., Caldwell, E.S., & Collier, A.C. (2000). Why don't patients and physicians talk about end of life care?: Barriers to communication for patients with acquired immunodeficiency syndrome and their primary care physician. *Archives of Internal Medicine, 160*(11), 1690–1696.

Cutilli, C.C., & Bennett, I.M., (2009). Understanding the Health Literacy of America Results of the National Assessment of Adult Literacy. *Orthopaedic Nursing 28*(1): 27–34.

Czaja, S.J., & Lee, C.C. (2007). The human computer-interaction handbook. In J. A. Jacko, & A. Sears (Eds.), *Information Technology and Older Adults* (2nd ed., pp. 777–792). New York: Lawrence Erlbaum.

Davies, K. (2006). What is effective intervention? Using theories of health promotion. *British Journal of Nursing, 15*(5), 252–256.

Davis, P.M., (1991). *Cognition and learning: A review of the literature with reference to ethnolinguistic minorities.* Dallas, TX: Summer Institute of Linguistics.

Davis, T.C., & Wolf, M.S. (2006). Literacy and misunderstanding prescription drug labels. *Annuals of Internal Medicine, 145*(12), 887–894.

Davis, T.C., Berkel, H.J., Arnold, C.L., Nancy, I., Jackson, R.H., & Murphy, P.W. (1998). Intervention study to increase mammography utilization in public health. *Journal of General Internal Medicine, 13*(4), 230–233.

Davis, T.C., Jackson, R.H., George, B.D., Long, S.W., Murphy, P.W., & Mayeaux, E.J.,…Truong, T. (1993). Reading ability in patients in substance misuse treatment centers. *International Journal of the Addictions, 28*(6), 571–582.

DeBrantes, F., Rastogi, A., & Painter, M. (2010). Reducing Potentially Avoidable Complications in Patients with Chronic Diseases: The Prometheus Payment Approach Reducing Potentially Avoidable Complications. *Health Services Research, 45*(6p2), 1854–1871

Deccache, A., & Aujoulat, I. (2001). A European perspective: Common developments, differences and challenges in patient education. *Patient Education and Counseling, 44*(1), 7–14.

DeGregori, T.R. (2003, July 17). *Health Issues.* Retrieved from American Council on Science and Health, December 10, 2011: http://www.acsh.org/healthissues/newsID.578/healthissue_detail.asp

Demetriou, A., & Raftopoulos, A. (Eds.). (2005). Cognitive developmental change: Theories, models and measurement. *Cambridge Studies in Cognitive and Perceptual Development.* Cambridge University Press. doi:10.1002/acp.1233

DeWalt, D.A., Berkman, N.D., Sheridan, S., Lohr, K.N., & Pignone, M.P. (2004). Literacy and health outcomes: A systematic review of the literature. *Journal of General Internal Medicine, 19*(12), 1228–1239.

Dewey, J. (1933). *How we think.: A restatement of the relation of reflective thinking to the educative process.* Chicago, IL: DC Heath Publishing.

Deyo, R.A., & Diehl, A.K. (1986). Patient satisfaction with medical care for low back pain. *Spine, 11*(1), 28–30.

Doak, C.C., Doak, L.G., & Root, J.H. (1995). *Teaching patients with low literacy skills.* Philadelphia, PA: J.B. Lippincott.

Dogra, N., Betancourt, J.R., Park, E.R., & Sprague-Martinez, L. (2009). The relationship between drivers and policy in the implementation of cultural competency training in health care. *Journal of the National Medical Association, 101*(2), 127–133.

Dube, L., Belanger, M.C., & Trudeau, E. (1996). The role of emotions in health care satisfaction. *Journal of Health Care Marketing, 16*(2), 45–51.

Durso, F.T., Nickerson, R.S., Dumais, S.T., Lewandowsky, S., & Perfect, T.J. (2007). *Handbook of Applied Cognition*. Wiley. Retrieved from http://lib.myilibrary.com/Browse/open.asp?ID=83871&loc=178

Eddy, J.D. (2007). Sequential Retrieval and Inhibition of Parallel (Re)Activated Representations: A Neurocomputational Comparison of Competitive Queuing and Resampling Models. *Adaptive Behavior, 15*(1), 51–71.

Edmunds, M. (2005). Health literacy: A barrier to patient education. *Nurse Practitioner, 30*(3), 54.

Ellis, S.E., Speroff, T., Dittus, R.S., Brown, A., Pichert, J.W., & Elasy, T.A. (2004). Diabetes patient education: A met-analysis and meta-regression. *Patient Education and Patient Counseling, 52*(1), 97–105.

Emaneul, E.J., & Goldman, L. (1998). Protecting patient welfare in managed care: Six safeguards. *Journal of Health Politics, Policy and Law, 23*(4), 635–639.

Emerson, R.W., (1912) Journals of Ralph Waldo Emerson: with annotations. Cambridge, MA: Houghton Miffilin Company.

Engler, A.J. (2005). Maternal stress and the white coat syndrome: A case study. *Pediatric Nursing, 31*(6), 470–473. doi: 942797851

Epstein, R., Franks, P., Fiscella, K., Shields, C.G., Meldrum, S.C., Kravitz, R.L., Duberstein, P.R. (2005). Measuring patient-centered communication in patient-physician consultations: Theoretical and practical issues. *Social Science and Medicine, 61*(7), 1516–1528.

Erlen, J.A. (2004). Functional health literacy: Ethical concerns. *Orthopaedic Nursing, 23*(2), 151–153.

Escalante, C.P., Weiser, M.A., Manzullo, E., Benjamin, R., Rivera, E., Lam, T.,... Rolston, K. (2004). Outcomes of treatment pathways in outpatient treatment of low risk febrile neurropenic cancer patients. *Journal of Supportive Care in Cancer, 12*(9), 657–662.

Esposito, T.J., Luchette, F.A., & Gamell, R.L. (2006). Do we need neurosurgical coverage in the trauma center? *Advances in Surgery, 40*, 213–221.

Evans, M. (2004). Poor performance AHA suffers year-end loss for second year in row. *Modern Healthcare, 34*(38), 9.

Faden, R.R., Becker, C., Lewis, C., Freeman, J., & Faden, A.L. (1981). Disclosure of information to patients in medical care. *Medical Care, 19*(7), 718–733.

Fallowfield, L., & Jenkins, V. (1999). Effective communication skills are the key to good cancer care. *European Journal of Cancer, 35*(11), 1592–1597.

Falvo, D.R. (1994). *Effective patient education: A guide to increased compliance* (2nd ed.). Gaithersburg, MD: Aspen.

Falvo, D.R. (2004). Effective Patient Education: A guide to increased compliance. Sudbury, MA: Jones and Barlett.

Feldman, J., & McPhee, D. (2008). *The Science of Learning and the Art of Teaching.* Clifton Park, NY: Thomson.

Fishbein, M. (1963). An investigation of relationships between beliefs about an object and the attitude toward that object. *Human Relations, 16,* 233–240

Fishbein, M., & Ajzen, I. (1975). *Belief, attitude, intention, and behavior: An introduction to theory and research.* Reading, MA: Addison-Wesley.

Fitzgerald, J.T., Funnell, M.M., Hess, G.E., Barr, P.A., Anderson, R.M., Hiss, R.G., & Davis, R.K. (1998). The reliability and validity of a brief diabetes knowledge test. *Diabetes Care, 21*(5), 706–710.

Fox, S. (2006, October 29). *Pew internet and American life project online health search 2006* [White paper]. Retrieved from Pew Internet: http://www.pewinternet.org/PPF/r/190/report_display.asp

Freeman, S.R., & Chambers, K.A. (1997). Home health care: Clinical pathways and quality integration. *Nursing Management, 28*(6), 45–48.

Friberg, F., Andersson, E.P., & Bengtsson, J. (2007). Pedagogical encounter between nurses and patients in a medical ward—a filed study. *International Journal of Nursing Studies, 44*(4), 534–544.

Friberg, F., Bergh, A.L., & Lepp, M. (2006). In search of details of patient teaching in nursing documentation: An analysis of patient records in a medical ward in Sweden. *Journal of Clinical Nursing, 15*(12), 1550–1558.

Funnell, M.M., & Anderson, R.M. (2004). Empowerment and self-management of diabetes. *Clinical Diabetes, 22*(3), 123–127.

Furnee, C.A., Groot, W., & Maassen van den Brink, H. (2008). The health effects of education: A meta-analysis. *Journal of Public Health, 18*(4), 417–421.

Gabbay, M.B., Cowie, V., Kerr, B., & Purdy, B. (2000). Too ill to learn: Double jeopardy in education for sick children. *Journal of Royal Society of Medicine, 93*(3), 114–117.

Galanti, G. (2008). *Caring for Patients from Different Cultures.* Philadelphia, PA: University of Pennsylvania Press.

GAO. (2006). *MEDICARE Communications to Beneficiaries on the Prescription Drug Benefit Could Be Improved.* United States Government Accountability Office.

Gerteis, M., Edgman-Levitan, S., Daley, J., & Delbanco, T. L. (Eds.). (1993). *Through the Patient's Eyes: Understanding and Promoting Patient-Centered Care.* New York, NY: Jossey-Bass.

Gerteis, M., Edgman-Levitan, S., Daley, J., & Delbanco, T.L. (Eds.). (1993). Through the Patient's Eyes: *Understanding and Promoting Patient-Centered Care.* New York, NY: Jossey-Bass.

Gessner, B.A. (1989). Adult education: The cornerstone of patient teaching. *The Nursing clincs of North America, 24*(3), 589–595.

Ginsburg, P.B. (2004). Controlling health care cost. *The New England Journal of Medicine, 351*(16), 1591–1593.

Given, B.K. (2002). *Teaching to the Brain's Natural Learning Systems.* Alexandria, VA.: Association for Supervision and Curriculum Development.

Glanz, K., Rimer, B.K., & Viswanath, K. (2008). *Health behavior and health education: Theory, research, and practice* (4th ed.). San Francisco, CA: Jossey-Bass.

Glasgow, R.E., Funnell, M.M., Bonomi, A.E., Beckham, V., & Wagner, E.H. (2002). Self-management aspects of the improving chronic care breakthrough series: Implementation with diabetes and heart failure teams. *Annals of Behavioral Medicine, 24*(2), 80–87.

Glasson, J., Chang, E., Chenoweth, L., Hancock, K., Hall, R., & Hill-Murray, F., & Collier, L. (2006). Evaluation is a model of nursing care for older patients using participatory action research in an acute medical world. *Journal of Clinical Nursing, 15*(5), 588–598.

Green , L.W., Mercer, S.L., Rosenthal, A.C., Dietz, W.H., & Husten, C.G. (2003). Possible lessons for physician counselling from the progress in smoking cessation in primary care. In Elmadfa, L., Anklam, E., & Konig, J.S. eds., Modern aspects of nutrition: present knowledge and future perspectives, 56, 191–194, Basal, Switzerland: Karger Publishers.

Green, C.D. (1994). Cognitivism: Whose party is it anyway? *Canadian Psychology, 35*(1), 112–123.

Green, L.W, & Kreuter, M.W. (2005). *Health program planning, an educational and ecological approach* (4th ed.). New York, NY: McGraw Hill.

Green, L.W., (2002). Health belief model. In Lester Breslow (Ed.), *Encyclopedia of Public Health* (Vol. 2, pp. 526–528). New York, NY: Macmillan Reference.

Green, L.W., & Kreuter, M.W. (1991). *Health Promotion Planning: An Educational and Environmental Approach* (2nd ed). Palo Alto, CA: Mayfield Publishing.

Greenburg, D. (2001). A critical look at health literacy. *Adult Basic Education, 11*(2), 67–79.

Greenburg, L.A. (1991). Teaching children who are learning disabled about illness and hospitalization. *The American Journal of Maternal/Child Nursing, 16*(5), 260–263.

Greene, M.G., & Adelman, R.D. (2003). Physician-older patient communication about cancer. *Patient Education and Counseling, 50*(1), 55–60.

Griggs, T. (October, 2011). Communication Key to Patient Education. Louisiana Medical News, Retrieved from: http://www.louisianamedicalnews.com/mod/secfile/viewed.php?file_id=65

Gross domestic report: Third quarter 2009. (2009, December 22). (U.S. Department of Commerce). Retrieved January 18, 2010, from Bureau of Economic Analysis

National Economic Accounts: http://www.bea.gov/newsreleases/national/gdp/2009/pdf/gdp3q09_3rd.pdf

Guadagnoli, E., & Ward, P. (1998). Patient-participation in decision-making. *Social Sciences and Medicine, 47*(3), 329–339.

Guevara, J.P., Wolf, F., Grum, C.M., & Clark , N.M.,(2003). Effect of educational interventions for self-management of asthma in children and adolescents: systematic review and meta-analysis. *British Medical Journal, 326*(7402). 1308–1309.

Gustafson, D.H., Arora, N.K., Nelson, E.C., & Boberg, E.W. (2003). Increasing understanding of patient needs during and after hospitalization. *Joint Commission Journal on Quality and Safety, 27*(2), 81–92.

Hahn, S.R. (2009). Patient-centered communication to assess and enhance patient adherence to glaucoma medication. *Opthalmology, 116*(11), S37–S42.

Hall, J.A., Roter, D.L., & Katz, N.R. (1988). Meta-analysis of correlates of provider behavior in medical encounters. *Medical Care, 26*(7), 657–675.

Hamilton, N. (2005). Grief and bereavement: Coping with loss of a spouse. *Nursing and Residential Care, 7*(5), 214–216.

Hanchate, A.D., Ashe, A.S., Gazmarian, J.A., Wolf, M.S., & Paasche-Orlow, M.K. (2008). The demographic assessment for health literacy (DAHL): A new tool for estimating associations between health literacy and outcomes in national surveys. *Journal of General Internal Medicine, 23*(10), 1561–1566.

Hanks, G. (1994). The efffect of healthcare reform on academic medicals. *The International Journal of Radiation Oncology Biology Physics, 31*(4), 999–1004.

Harlan, L. (2007). Under Pressure. *Network Journal, 14*(7), 36. Retrieved from Ethnic NewsWatch (ENW). doi: 1367503711)Hilgard, E.R. (1988). Review of B.F. Skinner's *the behavior of organisms. Journal of the Experimental Analysis of Behavior, 50*(2), 283–286.

Harper, W. (2007). Teaching health literacy: Building a foundation for safer health care. *Focus on Patient Safety Newsletter, 10*(1), 5–6. Retrieved from http://www.npsf.org/rc/pubs/CA_2007_07_01.pdf

Harper, W., Cook, S., & Makoul, G. (2007). Teaching students about health literacy: 2 Chicago initiatives. *American Journal of Healthy Behavior, 31*(Suppl. 1), S111–S114.

Health Canada (1999). *Toward a healthy future: Second report on the health of Canadians* [White paper]. Retrieved from Public Health Agency of Canada: http://www.hc-sc.gc.ca/hppb/phdd/report/text_versions/english/index.html

Health Canada. (1999). *Toward a healthy future: Second report on the health of Canadians.* Retrieved from http://www.hc-sc.gc.ca/hppb/phdd/report/text_versions/engllish/index.html

Health literacy in the United States. (2008). *Critical Care Nurse, 28*(4), 10.

Heisler, M., Bouknight, R.R., Hayward, R.A., & Smith, D.M. (2002). The relative importance of physician communication, participatory decision making, and patient understanding in diabetes self-management. *Journal of General Internal Medicine, 17*(4), 249–252.

Henderson, S. (2002). Influences on patient participation and decision-making in care. *Professional Nurse, 17*(9), 521–525.

Hernandez, P., Balter, M., Bourbeau, J., & Hodder, R. (2009). Living with chronic obstructive pulmonary disease: A survey of patients' knowledge and attitudes. *Respiratory Medicine, 103*(7), 1004–1012.

Hess, T.M., & Tate, C.S. (1991). Adult age differences in explanations and memory for behavioral information. *Psychology and Aging, 6*(1), 86–92.

Hesse, B.W., Nelson, D.E., Kreps, G.L., Croyle, R.T., Arora, N.K., Rimer, B.K., & Viswanath, K. (2005). Trust and sources of health information: The impact of the Internet and its implications for health care providers: Findings from the first Health Information National Trends Survey. *Archives of Internal Medicine, 165*(22), 2618–2624.

Hiemstra, R., & Sisco, B. (1990). *Individualizing Instruction.* San Francisco, CA: Jossey-Bass.

Higbee, H.L. (2001). *Your Memory: How it Works and How to Improve it.* New York: Da Capo Press.

Hilgard, E.R. (1988). Review of B F Skinner's the behavior of organisms. *Journal of the Experimental Analysis of Behavior, 50*(2), 283–286.

Hill, A., McPhail, S., Hoffmann, T., Hill, K., Oliver, D., Beer, C.,...Haines, T.P. (2009). A randomized trial comparing digital video disc with written delivery of falls prevention education for older patients in hospitals. *Journal of Geriatric Society, 57*(8), 1458–1463.

Hill, E.K. (2005). Assessing health literacy: Providing useable health information for seniors at discharge in northern Idaho. *Journal of Hospital Librarianship, 5*(4), 11–24.

Hill, R., & Dunbar, R. (2002). Social network size in humans. *Human Nature, 14*(1), 53–72.

Hirsch, E.D. (1988). *Cultural literacy: What every American needs to know.* New York: Vintage Books.

Hoare, C. (2006). *Handbook of adult development and learning.* New York, NY: Oxford University Press.Jensen, E. (2000). *Brain-based learning.* Thousand Oaks, CA; Corwin Press.

Hoffman, T., & McKenna, K. (2006). Analysis of stroke patients' and carers' reading ability and the content and design of written materials: Recommendations for improving written stroke information. *Patient Education and Counseling, 60*(3), 286–293.

Houts, P.S., Bachrach, R., Witmer, J.T., Tringali, C.A., Bucher, J.A., & Localio, R.A. (1998). Using pictographs to enhance recall of medical instructions. *Patient Education and Counseling, 35*(2), 83–88.

Houts, P.S., Witmer, J.T., Egeth, H.E., Loscalzo, M.J., & Zabora, J.R. (2000). Using pictographs to enhance recall of medical instructions II. *Patient Education and Counseling, 43*(3), 231–232.

Hoving, C., Visser, A., Mullen, P.D., van den Borne, B. (2010) A history of patient education by health professionals in Europe and North America: From authority to shared decision making education. *Patient Education and Counseling, 78*(3), 275–281.

Howard, D.H., Gazmararian, J., & Parker, R.M. (2005). The impact of low health literacy on the medical costs of Medicare managed care enrollees. *The American Journal of Medicine, 118*(4), 371–377.

Howard, D.H., Sentell, T., & Gazmararian, J.A. (2006). Impact of health literacy on socioeconomic and racial differences in health in an elderly population. *Journal of General Internal Medicine, 21*(8), 857–861.

Hutchinson, T.A., Hutchinson, N., & Arnaert, A. (2009). Whole person care: Encompassing the two faces of medicine. *Canadian Medical Association Journal, 180*(8), 845–846.

Hwang, S.W., Tram, C.Q., & Knarr, N. (2005). The effect of illustrations on patient comprehension of medication instruction labels. *BMC Family Practice, 16*(6), 26–32.

Iacono, J., & Campbell, A. (1997). *Patient and Family Education: The Compliance Guide to JCAHO Standards.* Marblehead, MA: HCpro.

Institute of Medicine of the National Academies. (2009). *Toward Health Equity and Patient-Centeredness: Integrating Health Literacy, Disparities Reduction, and Quality Improvement.* Washington, D.C.: The National Academies Press.

Institute of Medicine. (2002) Committee on Communication for Behavior Change in the 21st Century. *Speaking of Health: Assessing Health Communication Strategies for Diverse Populations.* Washington, DC: National Academies Press.

Jenkins, V., & Fallowfield, L. (2002). Can communication skills training alter physicians' beliefs and behavior in clinic? *Journal of Clinical Oncology, 20*(3), 765–769.

Jenkins, V., Fallowfield, L., & Saul, J. (2001). Information needs of patients with cancer: Results from a large study in UK cancer centres. *British Journal of Cancer, 84*(1), 48–51.

Jensen, E. (2000). *Brain-Based Learning: The New Science of Teaching and Learning.* Thousand Oaks, CA: Corwin Press.

Jervey, G.M. (2001, April). *American Medical Association Journal of Ethics.* Retrieved from Virtual Mentor: http://virtualmentor.ama-assn.org/2001/04/prsp1-0104.html

Johannessen, B. (2010). One Answer to Louisiana's Poor Health Rankings. Retrieved on December 12, 2011 from: http://www.lhcrmedicare.org/CareTransitionsInnovationAward.html

Jones, F. (2000). *Tools for Teaching.* Santa Cruz, CA: Fredric Jones & Associates.

Jones, S., & Fox, S. (2009, January 28). *Pew Research Center.* Retrieved from Pew Internet: http://pewinternet.org/Reports/2009/Generations-Online-in-2009.aspx

Karpf, M., Lofgren, R., & Perman, J. (2009). Health care reform and its potential impact on academic medical centers. *Academic Medicine, 84*(11), 1472–1475.

Kasmael, P., Atrkar-Roushan, Z., Majlesi, F., & Joker, F. (2008). Mother's knowledge about acute rheumatic fever. *Paediatric Nursing, 20*(9), 32–34.

Kaufman, J. (2008). Patients as partners. *Nursing Management, 39*(8), 45.

Kaye, M. (2009). *Health literacy and informatics in the geriatric population: The challenges and opportunities.* Retrieved from Online Journal of Nursing Informatics: http://ojni.org/13_3/Kaye.pdf

Kerr, M. (2008, July 22). Do I have white coat syndrome? *Irish Times,*16. doi: 1514464341

Kessels, R.P. (2003). Patients' memory for medical information. *Journal of the Royal Society of Medicine, 96*(5), 219–222.

Keulers, B.J., Schelting, M.R., Houterman, S., Van Der Wilt, G.J., & Spauwen, P.H. (2008). Surgeons underestimate their patients' desire for preoperative information. *World Journal of Surgery, 32*(6), 964–970.

Kick, E. (1989). Patient teaching for elders. *The Nursing clinics of North America, 24*(3), 681-686.

Kickbusch, I.S. (2001). Health literacy: Addressing the health and education divide. *Health Promotion International, 16*(3), 289–297.

Kindelan, K., & Kent, G. (1987). Concordance between patients' information preferences and general practitioners' perceptions. *Psychology and Health, 1*(4), 399–409.

Kinnersley, P., Edwards, A., Hood, K., Ryan, R., Prout, H., & Cadbury, N.,… Butler, C. (2008). Interventions before consultations to help patients address their information needs by encouraging question asking: Systematic review. *British Medical Journal, 337*(7662), 335–339.

Kirsch, S., Jungeblut, A., Jenkins, L., & Kolstad, A. (2002, April). *Adult literacy in America: A first look at the findings of the National Adult Literacy Survey* (NCES 1993–275). Retrieved from National Center for Educational Statistics: http://nces.ed.gov/pubs93/93275.pdf

Kirscht, J.P., Haefner, D.P., Kegeles, S.S., & Rosenstock, I.M. (1966). A national study of health beliefs. *Journal of Health and Human Behavior, 7*(4), 243–254.

Klein, S.B. (2009). *Learning Principles and Applications* (5 ed.). Thousand Oaks, CA: Sage.

Knowles, M.S. (1950). *Informal Adult Education: A Guide for Administrators, Leaders, and Teachers.* New York, NY: Association Press.

Knowles, M.S. (1968). Andragogy, not pedagogy. *Adult Leadership, 16*(10), 350–352, 386.

Knowles, M.S. (1973). *The adult learner: A neglected species.* Houston: Gulf Publishing.

Knowles, M.S. (1975). *Self-directed learning: A guide for learners and teachers.* Englewood Cliffs, NJ: Prentice Hall/Cambridge.

Knowles, M.S. (1977). *The adult education movement in the United States.* Malabar, FL: Krieger.

Knowles, M.S. (1980). *The modern practice of adult education: From pedagogy to andragogy.* Englewood Cliffs, NJ: Prentice Hall/Cambridge.

Knowles, M.S. (1984). *Andragogy in action: Applying modern principles of adult education.* San Francisco, CA: Jossey-Bass.

Knowles, M.S. (1984). *The adult learner: A neglected species* (3rd ed.). Houston, TX: Gulf.

Knowles, M.S. (1990). *The adult learner: A neglected species* (4th ed.). Houston, TX: Gulf.

Knowles, M.S., Holton, E.F., & Swanson, R.A. (2005). *The Adult Learner: The Definitive Classic in Adult Education and Human Resource Development* (6th ed.). San Diego, CA: Elsevier.

Korsch, B.M., Gozzi, E.K., & Francis, V. (1968). Gaps in doctor-patient communication. *Pediatrics, 42*(5), 855–871.

Krathwohl, D.R., Bloom, B.S., & Masia, B.B. (1964). *Taxonomy of educational objectives book 2: Affective domain.* New York, NY: David McKay.

Kraut, J. (Ed.). (1981). *American Jurisprudence* (2nd ed., Vol. 61). Rochester, NY: The Lawyer's Cooperative.

Kravitz, R.L., Bell, R.A., Azari, R., Krupat, E., Kelly-Reif, S., & Thom, D. (2002). Request fulfillment in office practice: Antecedents and relationship to outcomes. *Medical Care, 40*(1), 38–51.

Kripalani, S., & Weiss, B.D. (2006). Teaching about health literacy and clear communication. *Journal of General Internal Medicine, 21*(8), 888–890.

Kripalani, S., Henderson, L.E., Chiu, E.Y., Robertson, R., Kolm, P., & Jacobson, T. (2006). Predictors of medication self-management skill in a low literacy population. *Journal of General Internal Medicine, 21*(8), 852–856.

Kübler-Ross, E. (1969). *On Death and Dying.* New York, NY: Macmillian.

Kübler-Ross, E., & Kessler, D. (2005). *On Grief and Grieving: Finding the meaning of Grief Through the Five Stages of Loss.* New York, NY: Simon and Schuster.

Kurashige, E.M. (2008, May/June). Health literacy: What are the organizational barriers and concerns?. *AAACN Viewpoint*, 3–4.

Lahaie, U. (2008). Is nursing ready for webquests? *Journal of Nursing Education*, 47(12), 567–570.

Lainscak, M., & Keber, I. (2005). Validation of self assessment patient knowledge questionaire for heart failure patients. *European Journal pf Cardiovascular Nursing*, 4(4), 269–272.

Lambrew, J.M. (2004). Numbers matter: A guide to cost and coverage estimates in health reform debates. *The Journal of law, medicine, and ethics*, 32(3), 446–453.

Lancaster, G.I., O'Connell, R., Katz, D.L., Manson, J.E., Hutchinson, W.R., Landau, C., Yonkers, K.A. (2009). The expanding medical and behavioral resources with access to care for everyone health plan. *Annals of Internal Medicine*, 150(7), 490–492.

Lefrancois, G. (1995). *Theories of human learning: Kro's report* (3rd ed.). Pacific Grove, CA: Brooks/Cole.

Lenhart, A., Simon, M., & Graziano, M. (2001). *The Internet and Education: Findings of the Pew Internet and American Life Project.* Washington, D.C.: Pew Internet and American Life Project.

Leonard, K.J., & Wilijer, D. (2007). Patient are destined to manage their care. *Healthcare Quarterly*, 10(3), 76–78.

Levinson, W., Gorawara-Bhat, R., & Lamb, J. (2000). A study of patient clues and physician responses in primary care and surgical settings. *Journal of the American Medical Association*, 284(8), 1021–1027.

Levinson, W., Gorawara-Bhat, R., Daeck, R., Egener, B., Kao, A., Kerr, C., ... Kemp-White, M. (1999). Resolving disagreements in the patient-physician relationship: Tools for improving communication in managed care. *Journal of the American Medical Association*, 282(15), 1477–1483.

Levy-Storms, L. (2008). Therapeutic communication training in long term care interventions: Recommendations for future research. *Patient Education and Counseling*, 73(1), 8–21.

Leydon, G.M., Boulton, M., Moynihan, C., Jones, A., Mossman, J., Boudioni, M., & McPherson, K. (2000). Cancer patients' information needs and information seeking behaviour: In depth study. *British Medical Journal*, 320(7239), 909–913.

Lidell, E., & Fridlund, B. (1996). Long-term effects of comprehensive rehabilitation programme after myocardial infarction. *Scandinavian Journal of Caring Sciences*, 10(2), 67–74.

Lineker, S.C., Bell, M.J., Wilkins, A.L. & Bradley,E.M. (2001). Improving the following short-term home-based physical therapy are maintained at one year for people with moderate to severe rheumatoid arthritis. *Journal of Rheumatology, 28,* 165–168.

Lineker, S.C., Bradley, E.M., Hughes, E.A., & Bell, M.J. (1997). Development of an instrument to measure knowledge in individuals with rheumatoid arthritis: The ACREAU rheumatoid arthritis knowledge inventory questionnaire. *Journal of Rheumatology, 24*(4), 647–653.

Lofgen, R., Karpf, M., Perman, J., & Higdon, C.M. (2006). The US health care systems is in crisis: Implications for academic medical centers and their missions. *Academic Medicine, 81*(8), 713–720.

London, F. (n.d.). *No time to teach? A nurse's guide to patient and family education.* Philadelphia, PA: Lippincott Williams and Wilkins.

Longtin, Y., Say, H., Leape, L.L., Sheridan, S.E., Donaldson, L., & Pittet, D. (2010). Patient participation: Current knowledge and application to patient safety. *Mayo Clinic Proceedings, 1,* 53–62.

Lord, T.R. (1997). A comparison between traditional and constructivist teaching in college biology. *Innovative Higher Education, 21*(3), 197–216

Lorenzen, B., Melby, C.E., & Earles, B. (2008). Using principles of health literacy to enhance informed consent process. *Association of Operating Room Nursing Journal, 88*(1), 23–29.

Lorig, K. (1992). *Patient Education: A Pratical Approach.* St. Louis, MO: Mosby Year Book.

Luker, K., & Caress, A.L. (1989). Rethinking patient education. *Journal of Advance Nursing, 14*(9), 711–718.

Lund, C.H., Carruth, A.K., Moody, K.B., & Logan, C.A. (2005). Theoretical approaches to motivating change: A farm family case example. *American Journal of Health Education, 36*(5), 279–285.

MacGregor, J.N. (1987). Short-term memory capacity: Limitation or optimization. *Psychological Review, 94*(1), 107–108.

Maeland, J., & Havik, O. (1987). Psychological predictors for return to work after a myocardial infarction. *Journal of Psychosomatic Research, 31,* 471–481.

Maeland, J.G., & Havik, O.E. (1987). Measuring cardiac health knowledge. *Scandinavian Journal of Caring Sciences, 1*(1), 23–31.

Maeland, J.G., & Havik, O.E. (1987). The effects of an in-hospital educational programme for myocardial infarction patients. *Scandinavian Journal of Rehabilitation Medicine, 19*(2), 57–65.

Maguire, P., Booth, K., Elliot, C., & Jones, B. (1996). Helping health professionals involved in cancer care acquire key interviewing skills- the impact of workshops. *European Journal of Cancer, 32*(9), 1486–1488.

Maguire, P., Fairbarin, S., & Fletcher, C. (1986). Consultation skills of young doctors: Benefits of feedback training in interviewing as students persist. *British Medical Journal, 292*(14), 1573–1576.

Maibach, E.W., Van Duyn, M.S., & Bloodgood, B. (2006, July). *A marketing perspective on disseminating evidence-based approaches to disease prevention and health promotion.* Retrieved December 8, 2011, from CDC: http://www.cdc.gov/pcd/issues/2006/jul/05_0154.htm

Major, G., & Homes, J. (2007). How do nurses describe health care procedures? Analysing nurse-patient interaction in a hospital ward. *Australian Journal of Advanced Nursing, 25*(4), 58–70.

Makelainen, P., Vehvilainen-Julkunen, K., & Pietila, A.M. (2008). A survey of rheumatoid arthritis patients self-efficacy. *Internet Journal of Advanced Nursing Practice, 9*(2), 6.

Makoul, G. (2003). The interplay between education and research about patient-provider communication. *Patient Education and Counseling, 50*, 79–84.

Makoul, G., Arnston, P., & Schofield, T. (1995). Health promotion in primary care: Physician-patient communication and decision making about prescription medications. *Social Science and Medicine, 41*(9), 1241–1254.

Mancuso, J.M. (2008). Health literacy: A concept/dimensional analysis. *Nursing and Health Sciences, 10*, 248–255.

Maniaci, M.J., Heckman, M.G., & Dawson, N.L. (2008, May). Functional health literacy and understanding of medications at discharge. *Mayo Clinic Proceedings, 83*(5), 554–558.

Manning, K.D., & Kripalani, S. (2007). The use of standardized patients to teach low literacy communication. *American Journal of Healthy Behavior, 31*(Suppl. 1), S105–S110.

Marcus, E.N. (2006) The Silent Epidemic—The Health Effects of Illiteracy. *New England Journal of Medicine, 355*(4): 339–341.

Markus, K. (1997). Issues in Ethics Home Page. Retrieved from Santa Clara University December 2011,: http://www.scu.edu/ethics/publications/iie/v8n1/advancedirectives.html

Marr, D. (1971). Simple memory: A theory for archicortex. *Philosophical Transactions of the Royal Society of London B, 262*(84), 23–81. doi: 10.1098/rstb.1971.0078

Mayer, G.G., & Villaire, M. (2007). *Health literacy in primary care: A clinician's guide* (ed.). New York, NY: Springer.

Mayer, R.E. (1987). *Educational psychology: A cognitive approach.* Boston, MA: Little Brown.

McIntosh, W., & Kubena, K. (1996). An application of the health belief model to reductions in fat and cholesterol intake. *Journal of Wellness Perspectives, 12*(2), 98.

McKenzie, J. (2000). Information needs of patients with cancer: Similar study had similar findings. *British Medical Journal, 321*(7261), 632.

McLaughlin, N. (2008). The 2008 greeders' cup: Distress in financial markets can be blamed on fiscal irresponsibility. *Modern Healthcare, 38*(38), 41.

McPhee, J.T., Asham E.H., Rohrer M.J., Singh M.J., Wong, G., Vorhies, R.W., Nelson, P.R., & Cutler, B.S.(2007).The Midterm Results of Stent Graft Treatment of Thoracic Aortic Injuries. *Journal of Surgical Research, 138*(2) 181–188.

Meek, R., Kelly, A., & Hu, X. (2009). Use of the Visual Analog Scale to rate and monitor severity of nausea in the emergency department. *Academic Emergency Medicine, 16*(12), 1304–1310.

Merriam, S.B., & Caffarella, R.S. (1991). *Learning in adulthood: A comprehensive guide.* New York, NY: Jossey Bass.

Miller, G.A. (1956). The magical number seven, plus or minus two: Some limits on our capacity for processing information. *Psychological Review, 63*(2), 81–97. Retrieved from http://psychclassics.yorku.ca/Miller/

Miller, N.H., Hill, M., Kottke, T., & Ockene, I.S. (1997). The multilevel compliance challenge: Reccommendations for a call to action. *Circulation, 95*, 1085–1090.

Miller, W.R., & Rollnick, S. (2002). *Motivational Interviewing: Preparing People to Change.* New York, NY: Guilford Press.

Minninger, J. (1997). *Total recall: How to maximize your memory power.* New York, NY: MJF Books.

Mitchell, G., Murray, J., & Hynson, J. (2008). Understanding the whole person: Life limiting illness across the life span. In G. Mitchell, *Palliative Care: A Patient-Centered Approach* (pp. 79–107). Oxon, U.K.: Radcliffe Publishing, Ltd.

Monachos, C.L. (2007). Assessing and addressing low health literacy among surgical outpatients. *AORN Journal, 86*(3), 373–383.

Mondale, S., & Patton, S.B. (2001). *The Story of American Public Education.* Boston, MA: Beacon Press.

Moons, P., DeVolder, E., Budts, W., DeGeest, S., Elen, J., Waeytens, K., & Gewillig, M. (2001). What do patients with congenital heart disease know about their disease, treatment and prevention of complications?: A call for structured patient education. *Heart, 86*(1), 74–80.

Mordiffi, S.Z., Tan, S.P., & Wong, M.K. (2003). Information provided to surgical patients verses information needed. *AORN Journal, 77*(3), 546–562.

Morrow, D.G., Weiner, M., Young, J., Steinley, D., Deer, M., & Murray, M.D. (2005). Improving medication knowledge among older adults with heart failure: A patient centered approach to instruction design. *The Gerontologist, 45*(4), 545–552.

Mullen, P.D., Simons-Morton, D.G., Ramfrez, G., Frankowski, F., Green, L.W., & Mains, D.A. (1997). A meta-analysis of trails evaluating patient education and counseling for three groups of preventive health behaviors. *Patient Education and Counseling, 32*(3), 157–173.

Murray, M.D., & Callahan, C.M. (2003). Improving medication use for older adults: An integrated research agenda. *Annuals of Internal Medicine, 139*(5), 425–429.

Myers, J., & Pellino, T. (2009). Developing new ways to address learning needs of adult abdominal organ transplant recipients. *Progress In Transplantation, 19*(2), 160–166.

Nasaw, D. (1979). *Schooled to Order: A social history of public schooling in the United States.* Oxford, U.K.: Oxford University Press.

National Health Expenditure Data. (2010, January 4). Retrieved from Centers for Medicare and Medicaid Services: http://www.cms.hhs.gov/NationalHealthExpendData/25_NHE_Fact_Sheet.asp

National League of Nursing (NLN). (1976). *Patient Education.* New York, NY: NLN.

National Patient Safety Foundation (n.d.). *Ask Me 3 Program.* Retrieved from http://www.npsf.org/askme3/for_patients.php

National Quality Forum. (2005). *Implementing a national voluntary consensus standard for informed consent* [Brochure]. Washington, D.C.: Author.

Noddings, N. (2006). Educational leaders as caring teachers. *School Leadership & Management, 26*(4), 339–345

Novak, J. (1998). *Learning, creating and using knowledge: Concept maps as teaching tools in schools and corporations.* Mahwah, NJ: Lawrence Erlbaum Associates.

Nutbeam, D. (2000). Health literacy as a public health goal: A challenge for contemporary health education and communication strategies into the 21st century. *Health Promotion International, 15*(3), 259–267.

Oliver, J.W., Kravtiz, R.L., Kaplan, S.H., & Meyers, F.J. (2001). Individualized patient education and coaching to improve pain control among cancer outpatients. *Journal of Clinical Oncology, 19*(8), 2206–2212.

Ong, L.M., Visser, M.R., Lammes, F.B., & de Haes, J.C. (2000). Doctor-patient communication and cancer patients' quality of life and satisfaction. *Patient Education and Counseling, 41*(2), 145–156.

Ormrod, J.E. (1999). *Human learning.* Upper Saddle River, NJ: Prentice Hall.

Ormrod, J.E. (2008). *Human learning* (5th ed.). Columbus, OH: Prentice Hall.

Osborn, C.Y., Weiss, B.D., Davis, T.C., Skripkauskas, S., Rodrique, C., Bass, P.F., & Wolf, M.S. (2007). Measuring adult literacy in health care: Performance of the newest vital sign. *American Journal of Health Behavior, 31*(1), 37–45.

Osborne, H. (2005). *Health literacy from A to Z: Practical ways to communicate your health message.* Sudbury, MA: Jones and Barlett.

Overskeid, G. (1995). Cognitivist or behaviorist—who can tell the difference? The case of implicit and explicit knowledge. *British Journal of Psychology, 86*(4), 517.

Paasche-Orlow, M.K., Parker, R.M., Gazmarain, J.A., Nielsen-Bohlan, L.T., & Rudd, R.R. (2005). The prevalence of limited health literacy. *Journal of General Internal Medicine, 20*(2), 175–184.

Paasche-Orlow, M.K., Schillinger, D., Greene, S.M., & Wagner, E.H. (2006). How health care systems can begin to address the challenge of limited literacy. *Journal of General Internal Medicine, 21*(8), 884–887.

Palazzo, M.O. (2009). Patient and Family Education in Critical Care. In P. Morton, & D. Fontaine (Eds.), *Critical Care Nursing: A Holistic Approach.* New York, NY: Lippincott Williams & Wilkins.

Parikh, N.S., Parker, R.M., Nurss, J.R., Baker, D.W., & Williams, M.V. (1996). Shame and health literacy: The unspoken communication. *Patient Education and Counseling, 27*(1), 33–39.

Parker, R.M., Ratzan, S.C., & Lurie, N. (2003). Health literacy: A policy challenge for advance high-quality health care. *Health Affairs, 22*(4), 147–153.

Pavlov, I.P. (1927). *Conditioned reflexes: An investigation of the physiological activity of the cerebral cortex.* Retrieved from *Classics in the History of Psychology:* http://psychclassics.yorku.ca/Pavlov/

Pawlak, R. (2005). Economic considerations of health literacy. *Nursing Economics, 23*(4), 173–180.

Pender, N.J., Murdaugh, C.L., & Parsons, M.A. (2002). *Assumptions and theoretical propositions of the health promotion model.* Retrieved from University of Michigan Web Site: http://www.nursing.umich.edu/faculty/pender/HPM.pdf

Penzo, J.A., & Harvey, P. (2008). Understanding parental grief as a response to mental illness: Implications for practice. *Journal of Family Social Work, 11*(3), 323–338.

Perry, L. (2006). Promoting evidence-based practice in stroke care in Australia. *Nursing Standard, 20*(34), 35–42

Peterson, S.J., & Bredow, T.S. (2009). *Middle range theories: Application to nursing research* (2nd ed.). Philadelphia, PA: Lippincott Williams & Wilkins.

Phillips, L.D. (1999). Patient education: Understanding the process to maximize time and outcomes. *Journal of Intravenous Nursing, 22*(1), 19–35.

Piaget, J. (1954). *The construction of reality in the child,* New York, NY: Basic Books.

Piaget, J. (1967). *Biology and Knowledge.* Chicago, IL: University of Chicago Press.

Piaget, J. (1977). *The Essential Piaget.* New York, NY: Basic Books.

Piaget, J. (1983). Piaget's theory. In P. Mussen (Ed.). *Handbook of Child Psychology.* 4(1). New York, NY: Wiley.

Piaget, J. (1995). *Sociological Studies.* London, U.K.: Routledge

Pickert, K (2010) The Unsustainable U.S. Health Care System, Time: Swampland Retrieved December 8, 2011 from: http://swampland.time.com/2010/02/04/the-unsustainable-u-s-health-care-system/

Pierce, P.F., & Hicks, F.D. (2001). Patient decisions making behavior: An emerging paradigm for nursing science. *Nursing Research, 50*(5), 267–274.

Piette, J.D., Heisler, M., & Wagner, T.H. (2004). Cost-related medication underuse. *Archives of Internal Medicine, 164*(16), 1749–1755.

Pignone, M., DeWalt, D.A., Sheridan, S., Berkman, N., & Lohr, K.N. (2005). Interventions to improve health outcomes for patients with low literacy: A systematic review. *Journal of General Internal Medicine, 20*(2), 185–192.

Piotrowski, N.A. (2005). *Psychology Basics.* Salem Press. Retrieved from http://lib.myilibrary.com/Browse/open.asp?ID=97041&loc=498

Polit, D.F., & Beck, C.T. (2006). *Essentials of nursing research: Methods, appraisal, and utilization* (6th ed.). Philadelphia, PA: Lippincott Williams and Wilkins.

Prasauskas, R. & Spoo, L. (2006). Literally Improving Patient Health Outcomes. *Home Health Care Management Practice, 18*(4), 270–327.

Price, D. (1893). *The advancement of learning by Francis Bacon.* U.K.: Cassell & Company.

Prilleltensky, I. (2005). Promoting well-being: Time for a paradigm shift in health and human services. *Scandinavian Journal of Public Health, 66*, 53–60.

Pring, R. (2004). The skills revolution. *Oxford Review Of Education, 30*(1), 105–116.

Prochaska, J.O. (2009). Flaws in theory or flaws in the study: A commentary on the effect of transtheorectical model based inventions on smoking cessation, *68*(3), 407–409.

Prochaska, J.O., & Velicer, W.F. (1997). The transtheoretical model of health behavior change. *American Journal of Health Promotion, 12*(1), 38–48.

Prossier, H., Almond, S., & Walley, T. (2003). Influences on GPs' decision to prescribe new drugs: The importance of who says what. *Family Practice, 20*(1), 61–68.

Quirk, M., Mazor, K., Haley, H., Philbin, M., Fischer, M., & Sullivan, K., Hatem, D. (2008). How patients perceive a doctor's caring attitude. *Patient education and counseling, 72*(3), 359–366.

Raczynski, J.M., & DiClemente, R.J. (1999). *Handbook of Health Promotion and Disease Prevention.* New York: Kluwer Academic/Plenum.

Ramey, C. (2005). Did God create psychologists in His image? Re-conceptualizing cognitivism and the subject matter of psychology. *Journal of Theoretical and Philosophical Psychology, 25*(2), 173–190. doi:10.1037/h0091258.

Rankin, S.H., & Stallings, K.D. (1996). *Patient education: Issues, principles, practices* (3rd ed.). Philadelphia, PA: Lippincott.

Rankin, S.H., & Stallings, K.D. (2001). *Patient Education: Issues, principles, practices* (4th ed.). Philadelphia, PA: Lippincott-Raven.

Rankin, S.H., Stallings, K.D., & London, F. (2005). *Patient Education in Health and Illness* (5th ed.). Philadelphia, PA: Lippincott Williams and Wilkins.

Raynor, D.K. (2008). Medication literacy in a 2-way street. *Mayo Clinic Proceedings, 83*(5), 520–522.

Redman, B.K. (2001). *The practice of patient education* (9th ed.). St. Louis, MO: Mosby.

Redman, B.K. (2003). *Measurement tools in patient education* (2nd ed.). New York, NY: Springer.

Redman, B.K. (2004). *Advances in Patient Education.* New York: Springer.

Redman, B.K. (2006). *The practice of patient education: A case study approach* (10th ed.). St. Louis, MO: Mosby.

Redman, B.K. (2008). When is patient education unethical? *Nursing Ethics, 15*(6), 813–820.

Reiser, S.J. (1981). *Medicine and the reign of technology.* Cambridge, MA: Cambridge University Press.

Rice, E.G., & Okun, M.A. (1994). Older readers' processing of medical information that contradicts their beliefs. *Journal of Gerontology, 49*(3), 119–128.

Roberts, K. (2004). Simplify, Simplify: Tackling health literacy by addressing reading literacy. *American Journal of Nursing, 104*(3), 118–119.

Robinson, J.H., Callister, L.C. , Berry, J.A. , Dearing, K.A., (2008), Patient-centered care and adherence: Definitions and applications to improve outcomes. *Journal of the American Academy of Nurse Practitioners, 20*(12), 600–607.

Roediger, H.L., & Karpicke, J.D. (2006). The power of testing memory: Basic research and implications for educational practice. *Perspectives on Psychological Science, 1*, 181–210.

Rogers, E.S., Wallace, L.S., & Weiss, B.D. (2006). Misperceptions of medical understanding in low-literacy patients: Implications for cancer prevention. *Cancer Control, 13*(3), 225-229.

Roland, J. (2008). Rationality and logic. *The Review of Metaphysics, 61*(3), 632–634.

Rolls, E.T., Horrak, J., Wade, D., & McGrath, J. (1994). Emotion-related learning in patients with social and emotional changes associated with frontal lobe damage. *Journal of Neurology, Neurosurgery and Psychiatry, 57*(12), 1518–1524.

Rosen, G. (1977). *Preventive medicine in the United State 1900–1975.* New York, NY: Prodist.

Rosenstock, I.M. (1966). Why people use health services. *Millbank Memorial Fund Quarterly, 44*(3), 94–127.

Rosenstock, I.M., Strecher, V.J., & Becker, M.H. (1988). Social learning theory and the health belief model. *Health Educator Quarterly, 15*(2), 175–183.

Ross. (2006). Psychology of learning and motivation: The advances in research and theory. *Psychology of Learning and Motivation* (Vol 46). San Diego, CA: Elsevier Science & Technology. Retrieved from http://lib.myilibrary.com/Browse/open.asp?ID=63595&loc=221

Roter, D.L. (1977). Patient Participation in the patient-provider interaction: The effects of patient question asking on the quality of interaction, satisfaction and compliance. *Health Education and Behavior, 5*(4), 281–315.

Roter, D.L., Satashefsky-Margalit, R., & Rudd, R. (2001). Current perspectives on patient education in the US. *Patient Education and Counseling, 44*(1), 79–86.

Rumelhart, D.E. & Ortony, A. (1977). The representation of knowledge in memory. In R.C. Anderson & R J. Speiro (Eds.), *Schooling and the acquisition of knowledge.* Hillsdale, NJ: Erlbaum.

Rumsey, S., Hurford, D.P., & Cole, A.K. (2003). Influence of knowledge and religiousness on attitudes toward organ donation. *Transplant Proceedings, 35*(8), 2845–2850.

Safran, D.G., Kosinski, M., Tarlov, A.R., Rogers, W.H., Taira, D.H., Lieberman, N., & Ware, J.E. (1998). The primary assessment survey: tests of data quality and measurement Weiner, S.J., Barnet, B., Chang, T.L., & Daaleman, T.P. (2005). Processes for effective communication in primary care. *Annals of Internal Medicine, 142*(8), S709–S714.

Sandars, J., & Esmail, A. (2003). The frequency and nature of medical error in primary care: Understanding the diversity across studies. *Family Practice, 20*(3), 231–236.

Santrock, J.W. (2007). Cognitive development approaches. In E. Barrosse (Ed.), *A Topical Approach to Life-Span Development* (pp. 225–230). New York, NY: Beth Mejia.

Santrock, J.W. (2008). *A Topical Approach to Life Span Development.* New York, NY: McGraw-Hill.

Saunders, W. (1992). The constructivist perspective: Implications and teaching strategies for science. *School Science and Mathmatics, 92*, 136–141.

Save the Children. (2000). *State of the world's mothers* (Save the Children). Westport, CT: Save the Children.

Schell, T.J. (1986). Cognitive conception of learning. *Review of Educational Research. 56*(4), 411–437.

Schillinger, D., Grumbach, K., Piette, J., Wang, F., Osmond, D., & Daher, C.,... Bindman, A.B. (2002). Association of health literacy with diabetes outcomes. *Journal of American Medical Association, 288*(4), 475–482.

Schwartz, L.M., Woloshin, S., Black, W.C., & Welch, H.G. (1997). The role of numeracy in understanding the benefit of screening mammography. *Annuals of Internal Medicine, 127*(11), 966–972.

Schwartzberg, J.G. (2002). Low health literacy: What do your patients really understand? *Nursing Economics, 20*(3), 145–147.

Schwartzenberg, J.G. (2007). Communication techniques for patients with low health literacy: A survey of physicians, nurses, and pharmacists. *American Journal of Health Behavior, 31*(Suppl. 1), 96–104.

Schwartzenberg, J.G., Corrett, A., VanGeest, J., & Wolf, M.S. (2007). Communication techniques for patients with low health literacy: A survey of physicians, nurses, and pharmacists. *American Journal of Health Behavior, 31*(Suppl. 1), 96–104.

Schwartzenburg, J.G., VanGeest, J., Wang, C., Gazmararian, J., Parker, R., Roter, D.,...Schillinger, D. (Eds.). (2005). *Understanding health literacy: Implications for medicine and public health* (ed.). United States: AMA Press.

Secretary's Advisory Committee on National Health Promotion and Disease Prevention. (2009, November 3). *US Department of Health and Human Services.* Retrieved from Developing Healthy People 2020 on December 5, 2011: http://www.healthypeople.gov/hp2020/Objectives/files/Draft2009Objectives.pdf

Seligman, H.K., Wang, F.F., Palacios, J.L., Wilson, C.C., Daher, C., Piette, J.D., & Schillinger, D. (2005). Physician notification of their diabetes patients' limited health literacy. *Journal of General Internal Medicine, 20*(11), 1001–1007.

Shanks, D.R. (2010). Learning from association to cognition. *Annal Review of Psychology, 61*(1), 273–301.

Shaw, S.J., Huebner, C., Armin, J., Orzech, K., & Vivian, J. (2009). The role of culture in health literacy and chronic disease screening and management. *Journal of Immigrant Minority Health, 11,* 460–467.

Shea, S.C. (2006). Is it reallt noncompliance? In S. C. Shea, *Improving Medication Adherence: How to Talk with Patients about their Medications* (pp. 33–48). Philadelphia, PA: Wolters Kluwer Health Inc.

Shuell, T.J. (1990). Phases of meaningful learning. *Review of Educational Research, 60*(4), 531–547.

Simonds, S.K. (1978). Health education: Facing issues of policy, ethics, and social justice. *Health Education Monographs, 6*(Suppl. 1), 18–27.

Simonton, D.K. (1985). Intelligence and personal influence in groups: Four non-linear models. *Psychological Review, 92*(4), 532–547.

Simpson, M., Buckman, R., Stewart, M., Maguire, P., Lipkin, M., & Novack, D. (1991). Doctor-patient communication: The Toronto consensus statement. *British Medical Journal, 303*(6814), 1385–1387.

Skelton, A.M. (1997). Patient education for the millennium: Beyond and emancipation?. *Patient Education and Counseling, 31*(2), 151–158.

Skevington, S.M., & Garro, L. (1995). *Psychology of Pain*. Oxford, England: John Wiley & Sons.

Skinner, B.F. (1966). Contingencies of reinforcement in the design of a culture. *Behavioral Science, 11*(3), 159–166.

Skinner, B.F. (1974). *About Behaviorism*. New York, NY: Random House.

Skinner, B.F. (1991). *The Behavior of Organisms*. Acton, MA: Copley Publishing.

Slavin, R.E. (1995). A model of effective instruction. *Educational Forum, 59*(2), 166–176.

Smart, J. (2008). *Disability, Society, and the Individual* (2nd ed.). Austin, TX: Pro-Ed.

Smith, N. (2011). Patient Education: Determining a patient's readiness to learn. CINAHL Guide. Retrieved December 10, 2011 from: https://ehis.ebscohost.com/eds/detail?vid=30&hid=6&sid=1ab87eff-78d2-40ef-a8b8-c9e0602cb4f8%40sessionmgr112&bdata=JnNpdGU9ZWRzLWxpdmU%3d#db=nrc&AN=5000

Smith, S.K., Dixon, A., Trevena, L., Nutbeam, D., & McCaffery, K.L. (2009). Exploring patient involvement in healthcare decision making across different education and functional health literacy groups. *Social Science and Medicine, 69*(12), 1805–1812.

Sorrell, J.M. (2006). Health literacy in older adults. *Journal of Psychosocial Nursing, 44*(3), 17–20.

Sousa, D.A. (2006). *How the Brain Learns*. Thousand Oaks, CA: Corwin Press.

Spath, P.L. (Ed.). (2008). *Engaging Patients As Safety Partners: A Guide for Reducing Errors and Improving Satisfaction*. Chicago, IL: Health Forum.

Speros, C. (2005). Health literacy: Concept analysis. *Journal of Advanced Nursing, 50*(6), 633–640.

Spiers, M.V., Kutzik, D.M., & Lamar, M. (2004). Variation in medication understanding among the elderly. *American Journal of Health-System Pharmacists, 61*(4), 373–380.

Spring, B. (2008). Health decision making: Lynchpin of evidence-based practice. *Medical Decision Making, 28*(6), 866–874.

Stableford, S., & Mettger, W. (2007). Plain language: A strategic response to the health literacy challenge. *Journal of Public Health Policy, 28*(1), 71–93.

Stewart, M. (2008, March 14). 5 Rights of Patient Education. *A prescription for patient education: Assessing patient needs*. Joint Commission Resources Audio Conferences.

Stewart, M. (2009, December 16). Becoming an expert in patient education. Baton Rouge, LA.

Stewart, M., Meredith, L., Brown, J.B., & Galajda, J. (2000). The influence of older patient-physician communication on health and health-related outcomes. *Clinics on Geriatric Medicine, 16*(1), 25–36.

Stewart, M.N. (2008, November 7). Testing, testing 1,2,3—Patient education outcomes. *A Prescription for Patient Education: Assessing Patient Needs*. Joint Commission Resources Audio Conferences.

Stewart, M.N. (2008, September 19). 5 rights of patient education. *Neural Perspectives Conference*. Oklahoma City, OK.

Sthapornnanon, N., Sakulbumrungsil, R., Theeraroungchaisri, A., & Watcharadamrongkun, S. (2009). Social Constructivist Learning Environment in an Online Professional Practice Course. *American Journal of Pharmaceutical Education, 73*(1), 1–8.

Stone, M.A., Pound, E., Pancholi, A., Farooqi, A., & Khunti, K. (2005). Empowering patient with diabetes: A qualitative primary care study focusing on South Asians in Leichester, UK. *Family Practice, 22*(6), 647–652.

Stonecypher, K. (2009). Creating a patient education tool. *The Journal of Continuing Education in Nursing, 40*(10), 462–467.

Stuart-Hamilton, I. (2006). *The Psychology of Ageing: An Introduction*. London, U.K.: Jessica Kingsley Publishers. Retrieved from http://lib.myilibrary.com/Browse/open.asp?ID=92944&loc=102

Sudore, R. & Schillinger, D. (2009). Interventions to improve care for patients with limited health literacy. *Journal of Clinical Management, 16*(1), 20–29.

Sudore, R.L., Mehta, K.M., Simonsick, E.M., Harris, T.B., Newman, A.B., & Satterfield, S.,...Yaffe, K. (2006). Limited literacy in older people and disparities in health and healthcare access. *Journal of American Geriatrics Society, 54*, 770–776.

Sullivan, M. (2003). The new subjective medicine: Taking the patient's point of view on health care and health. *Social Science and Medicine, 56*(7), 1595–1604.

Swanson, L. (2007). New mental health services for deaf patients. *Canadian Medical Association Journal, 176*(2), 160.

Syred, M.E. (1981). The abdication of the role of health education by hospital nurses. *Journal of Advanced Nursing, 6*(1), 27–33.

Take steps now to reduce readmissions, ED visits within 30 days. (2009). *Hospital Case Management, 17*(5), 65–67.

Tang, P.C., & Lansky, D. (2005). The missing link: Bridging the patient-provider health information gap. *Health Affairs, 24*(5), 1290–1295.

Tattersall, R. (1995). Patient education 2000: Take-home messages from this congress. *Patient Education and Counseling, 26*(3), 373–377.

The Joint Commission. (2007). *"What did the doctor say?:" Improving health literacy to protect patient safety* (The Joint Commission). Oakbrook Terrace, IL: Author

Thompson, L.A., Knapp, C.A., Saliba, H., Guinta, N., Shenkman, E.A., & Nackashi, J. (2009). The impact of insurance on satiafaction and family-centered care for CSHCN. *Pediatrics, 124*(Suppl 4), S407–S413.

Thorndike, E. (1932). *The Fundamentals of Learning*. New York, NY: Teachers College Press.

Thorndike, E.L. (1911). *Animal Intelligence: Experimental Studies*. New York, NY: Macmillan. Retrieved from http://books.google.com/books?id=LC7GeCzw0lQC

Thorndike, E.L., Bregman, E.O., Tilton, J.W., & Wood, Y.E. (1928). *Adult Learning*. New York, NY: Macmillan.

Tkacz, V.L., Metzgner, A., & Pruchnicki, M.C. (2008). Health literacy in pharmacy. *American Journal of Health System Pharmacist, 65*(10), 974–981.

Tokarz, K.A. (2009). Patient education and self-advocacy : Queries and responses on pain management; erythromelalgia. *Journal of Pain and Palliative Care Pharmacotherapy, 23*(3), 295–297.

Tooth, L., Clark, M., & McKenna, K. (2000). Poor functional health literacy: The silent disability for older people. *Australasian Journal on Aging, 19*(1), 14–22.

Towle, A. & Godolphin, W. (1999). Framework for teaching and learning informed shared decision making. Retrieved from BMJ on December 30, 2011 from: http//www.bmj.com/content/319/7212/766.extract

Trossman, S. (2010). Issues up close: Nurses promoting true health understanding through literacy. *American Nurse Today, 5*(9), 32–33.

Trostle, J. (1988). Medical compliance as an ideology. *Social Science and Medicine, 27*(12), 1299–1308.

Tuan, L.T. (2011). Matching and Stretching Learners' Learning Styles. *Journal Of Language Teaching & Research, 2*(2), 285–294.

Twanmoh, J.R., & Cunningham, G.P. (2006). When overcrowding paralyzes an emergency department. *Managed Care, 15*(6), 54–59.

U.S. Department of Health and Human Services (2008). *Health literacy improvement*. Retrieved from http://health.gov/communication/literacy/default.htm

U.S. Department of Health and Human Services. (1999). *Patient's bill of rights* [Press release]. Retrieved from http://www.hhs.gov/news/press/1999pres/990412.html

U.S. Department of Labor. (2001). *Statistics about people with disabilities and employment*. Retrieved from http://.www.dol.gov/odep/archives/ek01/stats.htm

Untersmayr, E., & Jensen-Jarolim, E. (2006). The effect of gastric digestion on food allergy. *Current Opinion in Allergy and Clinical Immunology, 6*(3), 214–219.

Van de Borne, H.W. (1998). The patient from receiver of information to informed decision-maker1. *Patient Education and Counseling, 34*(2), 89–102.

Veldtman, G.R., Matley, S.L., Kendall, L., Quirk, J., Gibbs, J.L., Parsons, J.M., Hewison, J., (2001). Illness understanding in children and adolescents with heart disease. *Western Journal of Medicine, 174*(3), 171–173.

Vernon, J.A., Trujillo, A., Rosenbaum, S., DeBuono, B. (2007). *Low Health Literacy: Implications for National Health Policy*. Washington, DC: George Washington University School of Public Health and Health Services.

Villaire, M., & Mayer, G. (2009). Health Literacy: The Low-Hanging Fruit in Health Care Reform. *Journal of Health Care Finance, 36*(2), 55–59.

Visser, A., Deccache, A., & Bensing, J. (2001). Patient education in Europe: United differences. *Patient Education and Counseling, 44*(1), 1–5.

Visser, A.P. (1996). *Patient education and counseling*: Rights, duties, critics and credits. Patient education and counseling, *28*(1), 1–3.

Wagner, E. (2004). Part 1: The chronic care model [Video]. Available from http://www.researchchannel.org/prog/displayevent.aspx?rID=3877&fID=345

Wagner, E.H., Austin, B.T., Davis, C., Hindmarsh, M., Schaefer, J., & Bonomi, A. (2001). Improving chronic illness care: Translating evidence into action. *Health Affairs, 20*(6), 64–78.

Waitzkin, H. (1984). Doctor-patient communication: Clinical implications of social scientific research. *Journal of the American Medical Association, 252*(17), 2441–2446.

Walford, S. & Alberti, K.G. (1985) Biochemical self-monitoring: promise, practice and problems. Contemporary issues in clinical biochemistry, 2, 200–213.

Watson, J.B. (1930). *Behaviorism* (Rev. ed.). New York, NY: WW Norton.

Watson, J.B., & Rayner, R. (1920). *Conditioned emotional reactions*. Retrieved from Classics in the History of Psychology: http://psychclassics.yorku.ca/Watson/emotion.htm

Webb, J., Davis, T.C., Bernadella, P., Clayman, M.L., Parker, R.M., Adler, D., & Wolf, M.S. (2008). Patient-centered approach for improving prescription drug warning labels. *Patient Education and Counseling, 72*(3), 443–449.

Weiner, S.J., Barnet, B., Chang, T.L., & Daaleman, T.P. (2005). Processes for effective communication in primary care. *Annals of Internal Medicine, 142*(8), S709–S714.

Weinman, J., Petrie`, K.J., & Moss-Morris, R. (1996). The illness perception questionnaire: A new method for assessing the cognitive representation of illness. *Psychology and Health, 11*, 431–435.

Weinstein, N.D., Rutgers, U., & Cook, C., (1993). Testing four competing theories of *health*-protective behavior. *Health Psychology, 12*(4), 324–333

Weiss, B.D. (2007) Health Literacy and Patient Safety: Help patients understand, 2nd ed., American Medical Association Foundation, Retrieved December 2, 2011 from: http://www.ama-assn.org/ama1/pub/upload/mm/367/healthlitclinicians.pdf

Weiss, B.D., Blanchard, J.S., McGee, D.L., Hart, G., Warren, B., Burgoon, M., & Smith, K.J. (1994). Illiteracy among Medicaid recipients and its relationship to health care costs. *Journal of Health Care for the Poor and Underserved, 5*(2), 99–111.

White, J. (1999). Targets and systems of healt hcare costs control. *Journal of Health Politics, Policy, and Law, 24*(4), 653–696.

White, S. (2008). *Assessing the nation's health literacy: Key concepts and findings of the national assessment of adult literacy* (American Medical Association Foundation). Retrieved from AMA Foundation: http://www.ama-assn.org/ama1/pub/upload/mm/367/hl_report_2008.pdf

White, S., Chen, J., & Atchison, R. (2008). Relationship of preventative health practices and health literacy: A national study. *American Journal of Health Behavior, 32*(3), 227–242.

Whitehead, D. (2006). Health Promotion in the practice setting: Findings from a review of clinincal issues. *Worldviews on Evidence-based Nursing, 3*(4), 165–184.

Williams, A., Lindsell, C., Rue, L., & Blomkalns, A. (2007). Emergency department education improves patient knowledge of coronary artery disease risk. *Preventive Medicine, 44*(6), 520–525.

Willshaw D.J., & Buckingham J.T. (1990). An assessment of Marr's theory of the as a temporary memory store. *Philosophical Transactions: Biological Sciences, 329*(1253), 205–215.

Wingate, S. (1990). Patient perceptions of teir learning needs. *Dimensions of Critical Care Nursing, 9*(2), 112–118.

Wisconsin Public Health. (2002). *Containing Wisconsin public health costs* (Wisconsin Public Health & Health Policy Institute Brief). Wisconsin: Wisconsin Public Health.

Wlodkowski, R.J. (2008). *Enhancing Adult Motivation to Learn: A Comprehensive Guide for Teaching All Adults.* San Francisco, CA: John Wiley and Sons.

Wolf, M.S., Davis, T.C., Shrank, W., Rapp, D.N., Bass, P.F., & Connor, U.M.,… Parker, R.M. (2007). To err is human: Patient misinterpretations of prescription drug label instruction. *Patient Education and Counseling, 67*(3), 293–300.

Yancey, A., Tanjasini, S., Klein, M., & Tunder, J. (1995). Increased cancer screening behavior in women of color by culturally sensitive video exposure. *Preventive Medicine, 24*(2), 142–148.

Zins, J.E., Weissberg, P.P., Wang, M.E., & Walberg, H.J. (Eds.). (2004). *Building Academic Success on Social and Emotional Learning: What Does the Research Say?* New York: Teachers College Press.

Zull, J.E. (2006). Key Aspects of How the Brain Learns. In S. Johnson, & J. Taylor (Eds.), *The Neuroscience of Adult Learning: New Directions for Adult and Continuing Education* (110th ed., pp. 3–10). San Francisco, CA: Jossey Bass.

Index